Primary Care Interviewing

James Binder

Primary Care Interviewing

Learning Through Role Play

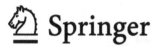 Springer

James Binder
Cabin Creek Health Systems
Dawes, WV, USA

Former Professor of Pediatrics
Marshall University School of Medicine
Huntington, WV, USA

Additional material to this book can be downloaded from http://www.springerimages.com/videos/978-1-4614-7223-0

ISBN 978-1-4614-7223-0   ISBN 978-1-4614-7224-7 (eBook)
DOI 10.1007/978-1-4614-7224-7
Springer New York Heidelberg Dordrecht London

Library of Congress Control Number: 2013938489

Printed on acid-free paper

Springer is part of Springer Science+Business Media (www.springer.com)

Foreword

It might mean something that when I searched the shelves in my office for a book with a "foreword" on which to model this one, what I found was a thin paperback by Gay Cheney titled, *Basic Concepts in Modern Dance*. In many ways, the two books—Cheney's and James Binder's—have a lot in common. They both set out to help students learn to use their bodies and their expressive capacities to relate to other people. They both recognize that it is possible to create a special space between people within which understanding and healing can take place. And they both recognize that this "art" is something that has to be methodically learned by observing demonstrations, practicing, getting feedback, and practicing some more. The dance studio has a wall of mirrors; in clinical education there are role plays.

We have long recognized that patient–clinician interactions are central to everything that medicine tries to accomplish. People looking for help have to be drawn into lasting treatment relationships, induced to divulge sensitive concerns, and supported while they decide what they want to do. But we have struggled to find efficient and replicable ways to teach and assess clinical interaction. Not everyone has access to standardized patients, or knows how to use audio or video feedback, despite the fact that we now all walk around with a miniature recording studio integrated with our telephones. Role plays are wonderful tools: they require no technology, they are infinitely flexible, and, in contrast to recordings, their "in the moment" nature makes them safe for learners at all levels.

The trouble with role play is that it takes skill to set one up and make it a good experience for one's students. That is where this book makes a lovely contribution. Built on long experience and well researched, it not only sets out a method but also walks the prospective leader through dozens of specific role plays for key situations encountered in primary care. One could put together a customized set of learning experiences for a particular rotation or continuing education workshop, or use one or two selectively with a learner who identified a particular area of need. I appreciate how much each chapter can stand independently as a teaching module and simultaneously as an instructor's guide and a student's handout.

In my professional lifetime, I have seen excitement about primary care rise and ebb and now rise again. At least for those of us of a certain age, it is hard to separate a vision of what primary care stands for from a larger belief that medicine is at its best when it reinforces our common humanity and the sense of mutual respect and responsibility we have for each other, patient and clinician, student and teacher. That belief suffuses Dr. Binder's book, and, even better, the book offers us a way to teach it.

Larry Wissow, MD, MPH
Professor, Department of Health, Behavior, and Society
John Hopkins School of Public Health
Baltimore, MD

Preface

A 10-year-old boy with high-functioning autism presents to the primary care clinic with a history of intermittent LUQ abdominal pain, present for several months. His mother, who suffers from a cognitive impairment, loudly demands an x-ray and an immediate referral to a specialist. After evaluating the child, the first-year resident presents the situation to the attending. The resident feels frustrated. The child has no red flags in the history or physical exam and he thinks an x-ray and referral are not warranted; yet, the mother is insistent. His diagnosis is GERD. The resident and attending discuss the family. People, who are demanding, like this mother, often have underlying intense anxiety. The attending makes a guess that the mother is imagining the cause of the illness to be more serious than is warranted. He suggests that he and the resident do a brief role play. The resident plays the distraught mother. The attending demonstrates basic interviewing techniques of empathic understanding and direct inquiry into the mother's theory of illness, which is likely driving her intense anxiety. The resident and attending switch roles. The whole role play takes 4 minutes. The resident then uses this approach with the mother and uncovers her fear that the pain means something is wrong with the child's heart. He reassures her that the child has a normal heart and simply has dyspepsia. The mother notes that the child has gained a lot of weight in the last year. She learns that may have contributed to the dyspepsia. She agrees to a trial of a proton-pump inhibitor with a follow-up visit in 3 weeks.

Primary care is complex, is unpredictable, and requires a biopsychosocial orientation. The case above is representative of how people present in primary care. They often present with common medical conditions that don't seem routine because of their unique personal and family contexts. Clinicians in primary care, many times, deal with problems that are not attributable to a specific diagnosis [1]. Even when the diagnosis is specific, as above, people present with needs, not diseases [2]. It is precisely these aspects of primary care that make role-playing ideally suited to teach clinicians how to interview and relate to patients. The actor-patient presents with a problem and he, she, or the family communicates with the interviewer about the problem or situation. Each person affects the response of the other in a dynamic way, mimicking the actual encounter that occurs in primary care. Flexibility, persistence, and attention to the person of the patient—essential qualities of a good primary care clinician—are learned through realistic enactments. In the above situation, the attending could have used any number of role-play approaches, depending on the resident's needs. For example, he could have asked the resident questions related to self-awareness to help the resident access his emotional reaction to the mother's loud demands and consider how to manage them during a brief role play. Role-playing can be quickly adapted to meet the unique needs of both the trainee and the patient. Role-playing is a person-centered approach, one of the four pillars of primary care identified by Barbara Starfield [3].

The sample role plays at the beginning of each chapter are created from my teaching experience to illustrate the teaching points. They are not representative of any specific trainee or role play situation from my teaching groups. Some of the role plays are available for viewing at: http://www.springerimages.com/videos/978-1-4614-7223-0.

Huntington, WV, USA   James Binder

References

1. Rosser WW. Approach to diagnosis by primary care clinicians and specialists: is there a difference. J Fam Pract. 1996;42:139–44.
2. American College of Physicians. How is a shortage of primary care physicians affecting the quality and cost of medical care? Philadelphia: American College of Physicians; 2008: White Raper (Available from American College of Physicians, 190 N. Independence Mall West, Philadelphia, PA 19106.)
3. Starfield B. Perspective: the future of primary care: refocusing the system. N Eng J Med. 2008;359:2087–91

Acknowledgements

I want to thank Fred Platt for his warmth, generosity, and knowledge—he has mentored me during the process of writing two books on medical interviewing. The format for my current book is modeled after *Field Guide to the Difficult Patient Interview* by Fred Platt and Geoffrey Gordon.

I want to give a special thanks to Susan McDaniel, Craig Bryan, and Vann Joines. Susan read many chapters in the book, offering her expertise and invaluable ideas. Craig reviewed the chapter on suicide assessment, making important suggestions for improvement. Vann taught me the importance of safety, affirmations, and humor in creating healthy relationships.

Richard Lansing, my editor, has kindly and patiently nurtured me through the process of writing this book.

The Joan C. Edwards School of Medicine's Department of Pediatrics and chairman, Joseph Werthammer, have encouraged my interest in interviewing and role play for many years. I have learned so much from the interviewing seminars for medical students and those for residents. Denise Smith helped me in my research on interviewing with an unfailing work ethic and consistently positive attitude.

Barbara Dallmann provided excellent technical support and a number of helpful comments about the manuscript itself. Allison Hartman, my copy editor, made this a stronger book with her skills and attention to detail.

Many of the ideas or topics in this book reflect the work of others in the field—I want to mention two of them. Shawn Shea has promoted and effectively used role-playing for teaching interviewing skills over the last several decades. During this same time period, the American Academy on Communication in Healthcare has been a powerful leader in the field of medical interviewing.

I want to acknowledge my family, Susan, James, Michael, Maura, and Daniel for their encouragement throughout the process of writing my second book. I consulted with my son Michael, who specializes in Internal Medicine, on adult clinical issues. He is a coauthor of chapter 11: *Across the Lifespan*. I am deeply grateful to my wife Susan for editing, supporting, and loving me throughout this project.

Huntington, WV, USA   James Binder

Contents

Part I Introduction

1 Personal Story 13
Role Play 13
Objectives 13
Feedback 14
Replay 15
Feedback 16
Obstacles to Teaching Personal Story 16
Strategies 16
Personal Story 16
Key Points 18
References 18

2 Contracting 21
Role Play 21
Objective 21
Feedback 22
Objective 22
Feedback 23
Replay 24
Feedback 24
Obstacles to Teaching Contracting 24
Strategies 25
Contracting 25
Psychosocial Issues 27
Mini contracts 28
One final note 29
Key Points 30
References 30

3   Open-Ended Inquiry..   31
    Role Play...   31
    Objectives..   31
    Feedback   32
    Objectives..   33
    Feedback   33
    Replay   34
    Obstacles to Teaching Open-Ended Inquiry   34
    Strategies...   34
    Open-Ended Inquiry..   35
    Create a Safe Environment   35
    Nonverbal Tools   36
    Practical Aspects of Formulating Open-Ended
    Questions and Facilitations..   37
    Incongruence Between Verbal and Nonverbal..   39
    Key Points   39
    References..   39

4   Affirmations..   41
    Role Play...   41
    Objectives..   41
    Feedback   42
    Replay   43
    Feedback   44
    Obstacles to Teaching Affirmations..   44
    Strategies...   44
    Affirmations   45
    Empirical Support for Affirmations   45
    Practical Points..   46
    Key Points   48
    References..   48

5   Eliciting and Responding to Emotions...   49
    Role Play...   49
    Objectives..   49
    Feedback   50
    Replay   50
    Feedback   51
    Objectives..   51
    Feedback   51
    Demonstration to Trainees   52
    Feedback   53
    Obstacles to Teaching Eliciting and Responding to Emotions   53
    Strategies...   53
    Eliciting and Responding to Emotions   53
    Direct Inquiry..   55

Indirect Inquiry 56
   Third-Person Technique.. 56
Clinician's Emotional Literacy 56
Responding to Patients' Feelings... 57
   Deepen Emotional Experience.. 58
Responding to Intense Fear or Sadness 59
   Fear 59
   Sadness.. 60
Closing the Window.. 60
Key Points 61
References.. 61

6 Uncovering Self-Diagnosis... 63
Role Play... 63
Objective 63
Feedback 64
Obstacles to Teaching Uncovering Self-Diagnosis..................................... 65
Strategies... 65
Uncovering Self-Diagnosis and Other Health Beliefs 65
Explanatory Model... 66
Key Points 68
References.. 69

7 Structure 71
Role Play... 71
Objectives.. 71
Feedback 72
Obstacles to Teaching Structuring 73
Strategies... 73
Structuring... 73
Tasks of Interview 74
   Opening Phase 74
   Middle Phase.. 74
   Concluding Phase... 74
Structuring Strategies... 74
   Preparation 75
   Use of Computers 75
   Time Management 75
Contract... 76
Make the Process Overt 76
Guiding 77
Structuring a Wandering Patient 79
Family 80
Key Points 81
References.. 81

8   Accuracy   83
      Role Play   83
      Objectives..   83
      Feedback   84
      Objective   85
      Feedback   86
      Replay   86
      Feedback   87
      Obstacles to Teaching Accuracy   87
      Strategies...   87
      Accuracy   88
      Clinician Interviewing Style   88
      Patients Who Are Vague   89
          Cognitive Deficit..   89
          Vagueness...   90
          Increasing Precision with Vague Patients   90
          Recall Errors   91
      Interviewing Tools for Sensitive Issues   91
          Normalization   91
          Gentle Assumption...   92
          Denial of the Specific..   92
          Behavioral Incident   93
      Key Points   93
      References   94

9   History of Present Illness..   95
      Role Play   95
      Objectives..   95
      Time Out   96
      Replay   96
      Feedback   97
      Objectives..   97
      Feedback   99
      Role Play: Front to Back (1&2)..   99
      Obstacles to Teaching History of Present Illness.............................   99
      Strategies... 100
      History of Present Illness 100
      Preliminary Work.. 100
          Secondary Data 101
      Primary Data... 101
      Focused Questions 102
          Onset and Chronology 104
          Position and Radiation 104
          Quality.. 104
          Quantification... 105

Related Symptoms 105
Setting 106
Transforming (Aggravating/Alleviating) Factors 106
Conversational Style 106
Clinical Context 107
Key Points 108
References 108

10 Concluding Phase 109
Role Play 109
Objectives 109
Replay 111
Feedback 112
Obstacles to Teaching Concluding Phase 112
Strategies 113
Concluding Phase 113
Key Points 117
References 117

11 Across the Life Span 119
James Binder and Michael Binder
Role Play 119
Objectives 119
Feedback 120
Objectives 121
Feedback 122
Replay 122
Feedback 123
Obstacles to Teaching Interviewing Across the Life Span 123
Strategies 123
Across the Life Cycle 124
Preschool Children 124
School-Aged Children 125
Adolescence 126
Interfering Cognitions 126
Set the Stage 126
Third Phase 127
Shut Down Adolescent 128
Geriatric Medicine 130
Comprehensive Assessment 130
Family Involvement 131
Other Barriers 131
Key Points 132
References 132

Part II   Teaching Complex Interviewing Skills

12   Family Concepts 137
   Level of Functioning 138
   Structure 139
   Family Process 140
     Differentiation 140
     Basic Belief About Okayness 140
     Stroking Pattern 140
     Family Mood 141
   Family Through Time 141
   Cultural Humility 142
   Clinical Level of Involvement 143
   Forms of a Family Visit 144
     Routine Family Office Visits 144
     Family Conference 146
     Think Family (with Individual Patients) 146
   References 147

13   Family Interviewing 149
   Role Play 149
   Potential Role Play Objectives 149
   Objectives 150
   Feedback 150
   Replay 151
   Feedback 152
   Objective 152
   Feedback 153
   Replay 153
   Macrotraining 154
   Objective 154
   Feedback 155
   Replay 156
   Obstacles to Family Role Plays 157
   Strategies 158
   Family Interviewing 158
     Rapport 158
     Organize/Contract 160
     Facilitate Discussion and Transmit Information 162
     Identify Strengths, Resources, and Supports 165
     Establish a Plan 165
   Key Points 166
   References 166

14 Mental Health.. 167
    Role Play... 167
    Objective (12–15-min Role Play) 167
    Feedback 169
    Obstacles to Assessing and Treatment of Mental Health
    Conditions During Training 170
    Strategies... 170
    Mental Health.. 170
    Identifying Mental Health Disorders 171
        Core Interviewing Skills 171
    Interview Skills Needed to Formulate a Good Differential Diagnosis 173
    Collaborative Family Health Care Model.. 174
    Mental Health Referral 176
    Key Points 177
    References.. 178

15 Body–Mind Integration 181
    Role Play... 181
    Objective 181
    Feedback 182
    Replay 182
    Feedback 183
    Obstacles to Teaching Body–Mind Integration 183
    Strategies... 183
    Body–Mind Integration.. 184
    Interviewing Strategies 185
        Negotiate a Mutually Acceptable Diagnosis............................. 185
        Invite the Family to Participate Early in Treatment.................. 186
        Affirm the Patient and Family's Strengths................................ 186
        Avoid Psychosocial Fixation... 187
        Judge Progress by Monitoring Changes in Functioning........... 187
    Key Points 187
    References.. 187

16 Suicide Assessment.. 189
    Role Play... 189
    Objectives.. 189
    Feedback 190
    Replay 192
    Feedback 192
    Objectives.. 193
    Feedback 196
    Objectives.. 197
    Feedback 197
    Obstacles to Teaching Suicide Assessment 198
    Strategies... 198

Suicide Assessment in Primary Care 198
Interfering Cognitions 198
Setting the Platform 199
Normalization 200
Database 201
Assess for Past Suicidal Behaviors 202
   Screen for Multiple Attempts and Assess Attempt History 203
Assess the Current Suicidal Episode 203
   Screen for Protective Factors 203
Means Restricting Counseling 204
Note 204
Key Points 205
References 205

17 Sex 207
Role Play 207
Objectives 207
Feedback 208
Replay 209
Feedback 209
Obstacles to Teaching Interviewing About Sex 210
Strategies 210
Sex 211
Self-examination for Interfering Cognitions 211
Setting the Stage 211
Adolescent Sexuality 215
Set the Stage 215
   Normalization 216
Key Points 217
References 217

18 Motivational Interviewing 219
Role Play 219
Objectives 219
Objectives 220
Feedback 221
Replay 222
Feedback 223
Obstacles to Teaching Motivational Interviewing 223
Strategies 223
Motivational Interviewing 223
Motivational Interviewing with Alcohol Use Disorders 224
   Self-examination 225
   Set the Stage 225
   Assessment 225
   CAGE 226

Validity 226
Complete the Assessment 226
Brief Interventions in Alcohol Use Disorders 227
Use the Elicit–Provide–Elicit Framework for Giving Information 227
Roll with the Resistance 228
Support Change 228
Give Specific Recommendations Congruent
with Expert Guidelines 229
Key Points 230
References 230

19 Giving Bad News 233
Role Play 233
Objectives 233
Feedback 234
Replay 235
Obstacles to Teaching Giving Bad News 236
Strategies 236
Giving Bad News 236
Staying Emotionally Present to Families 236
Practical Recommendations for Giving Bad News 237
Emotional Reaction 239
Key Points 240
References 241

20 Challenging Interviews 243
Role Play 243
Objectives 243
Feedback 244
Replay 245
Feedback 246
Objectives 247
Feedback 247
Replay 248
Replay 249
Feedback 249
Obstacles to Teaching Challenging Interviews 249
Strategies 250
Challenging Interviews 250
Contract 250
Empathic Communication 251
Meaning of Illness or Problem 252
Include Family 253
Key Points 253
References 254

Appendix A 255

Appendix B 257

Glossary of Interviewing Terms.. 259

Index... 263

Part I
Introduction

The patient interview is the core of clinical medicine. Being a good primary care practitioner takes an ability to interview and manage interviews well. It is the most utilized skill in primary care. Learning to interview well requires no less practice than that required to master a musical instrument or learn to play a new sport. Role-play methods have a unique ability to address the multiple, complex, and unpredictable demands of learning to interview in primary care.

Role-Playing Benefits

Role-playing has strong benefits for teaching interviewing skills.

1. The most important is the ability to assess a trainee's skills accurately [1]. Trainee self-report of physician–patient encounters can be misleading due to a lack of awareness of nonverbal communication and other behaviors impacting the interview.
2. It has broad clinical applicability (e.g., obtain a history of present illness, discuss weight loss, ask about sexual behaviors, deal with an angry patient, perform a family interview, and give bad news), which is a major advantage over other teaching methods, such as direct observation.
3. Role-playing lends itself to the repetition needed for consolidation of interviewing skills. Consolidation of skills leads to confidence and a sense of competence [1].
4. Faculty members can readily model a multitude of interviewing techniques based on the immediate needs of the trainee [1]. A brief role play takes only 3–4 min.
5. Role-playing is evidence based and a key element of microcounseling.[1] A meta-analysis of 81 empirical studies of microcounseling found it to be an effective educational method [2]. Furthermore, acquisition of the three basic skills

---

[1]Microcounseling is a methodology for teaching basic counseling skills created by Allen Ivey in the 1960s.

of attending, paraphrasing, and reflection correlated with enhanced empathy (a complex skill) [3].

6. And, it is fun! Laughter is a common outcome of group role plays. This is no small benefit for medical students and residents undergoing strenuous training.

Barriers to Role Play

Trainee anxiety constitutes the main obstacle to setting up a role play. This is normal and to be expected. Medical students and residents have been successful at most endeavors they have tried throughout their lives. Typically, this has not included developing expertise in interpersonal communication. Making interview 'errors,' which are immediately apparent to peers and mentor, can feel vulnerable to trainees [1]. A supportive, organized approach is needed to help them with that vulnerability.

In our Marshall University first-year resident interviewing group, we spend time learning the participants' personal stories and joining with them. Once joining has occurred—and this is not rushed—trainees receive information about role-playing. It is important for them to understand how they will benefit in the long run by challenging themselves to do role plays. This education occurs over time. Trainees initially observe a faculty member role play. Trainees are then started on very basic role plays so that success is almost guaranteed [4].

A second objection needs to be directly addressed. Participants may believe that the role play is not real—that it is fake or phony. However, both the interviewer and interviewee are real people having real interactions. The interactions represent what truly happens with actual patients. It is possible that an interviewer might initially interact differently in role play than he or she does with patients. Making the role play as realistic as possible addresses that problem. In my experience, the unnaturalness fades quickly. If they remain skeptical, trainees can be asked to experiment with the process for a specified time period. Invariably this problem resolves itself.

Practical Aspects of Role-Playing

Agreement on a contract for role-playing allows each participant to take responsibility for his or her own part, setting the stage for a successful educational experience. A clear contract supports an emotionally safe process by specifying what the participants agree to do, how long it will take, what the outcome of the process will be, and how everyone will know that the goals of the exercise have been reached. Trainees who have had negative experiences with role plays may be reluctant to participate [1]. Resistance is made overt so it can be dealt with in an open and honest discussion.

Faculty:	What experiences have you had with role playing in the past?
Trainee #1:	I was at a workshop in college. I just wanted to observe. The leader coerced me into participating in a role play. I was sweating and felt very embarrassed.
Faculty:	That's too bad that you had such a painful experience. It sounds like you participated in a role play in which safe guidelines were not established. We will talk about how role plays can be made safe.
Trainee #1:	Good. I think that is important.
Faculty:	Let me go over how the role plays will be set up. We will start with basic skills such as attending, listening, and making a reflective statement. Later, we will move to complex skills. I will demonstrate the technique first and repeat it if anybody wants to see the skill again. We will establish 1–2 objectives for each role play, which will be done realistically in order to get the most benefit from the exercise. An interviewer can call a time out at any point to ask for suggestions. All members of the group agree to mentally participate by actively observing. Does anybody have questions?
Trainees:	(no response)
Faculty:	After the role play, we will give affirmations regarding what we thought went well. This will include comments from the interviewing participants. I will then ask everyone for any options they have for doing the interview differently. Feelings can arise during a role play. They may be related to current issues in the interviewer's life or even his or her family of origin. The opportunity to process those feelings is one of the advantages of role playing in a group. It is important that all members agree to confidentiality so that people feel free to talk. Does everyone agree?
Trainees:	Yes.
Faculty:	There is one more thing. In my experience it works best if I call on different participants to do a role play, rather than ask for volunteers. Of course, the person is free to decline. Is this okay with everyone?
Trainees:	Yes.

It is not unusual for trainees to be reluctant and to need time for role-playing to feel safe and useful. Occasionally, a trainee will have an intense, even phobic reaction. The mentor can meet individually with such a student and devise a different curriculum for learning interviewing, perhaps involving didactics and observation [1].

As noted above, it is important to have an organized plan when teaching interviewing skills with role play. Shawn Shea and Christine Barney describe an approach that is practical, safe, and effective [1, 4]. Role plays in this text are patterned after their method.

Role Plays in this Text will have the Following Characteristics:

1. The initial, basic interviewing skills that will be role played are defined behaviorally. Example of a role-play objective: Trainee will demonstrate a gentle command as a way to invite the patient to talk. A gentle command is defined as a statement beginning with 'tell me' or 'describe,' and said with a gentle voice, such as, 'tell me all about the cough' [5].

2. The basic skills are practiced until they have been overlearned. Initially, approximations to the skill are accepted [1]. Recently acquired techniques are practiced along with new skills being learned so that skills are maintained. The skills are practiced with some variations so they are generalized and consolidated [1, 4]. Complex sequences (such as those included within family interviews, sensitive interviews, giving bad news, etc.) follow the acquisition of a series of basic skills. All skills must be demonstrated in order to show mastery.

3. Objectives are established for each role play and written down on a flipchart so that the role play is focused and tight. Trainees and faculty negotiate the objectives before starting a role play.

4. Role-playing the patient or family is done realistically. This establishes the credibility and usefulness of the technique being learned. A good way to make the role play realistic is for the actor to think of a specific patient, including the nonverbal mannerisms of that patient [1].

5. Trainees role-playing a patient are invited to "be the patient," or "be the mom." When trainees allow themselves to experience the patient position, they can better appreciate the power of a specific interviewing technique. This may increase their motivation to use the technique in their own clinical practice [1]. In a similar manner, a trainee, having a difficult time empathizing with a patient, can be invited to switch chairs and play the part of the patient. Sometimes this enhances his or her ability to imagine what it is like being the patient or family member.

   A trainee appears to be having difficulty demonstrating an empathic summary with a mother of a drug addicted baby during a role play. The faculty member takes a time out and asks the trainee what he is experiencing. The trainee feels judgmental and frustrated with the mother. He agrees to experiment being the mother while the faculty member asks the mother her personal story. The group chuckles briefly as the trainee plays the mother. However, after 3–4 minutes, the role play is completed. The trainee states he is better able to imagine what it is like being the drug addicted mother, who is experiencing anxiety and guilt. He returns to the role of interviewer and makes a genuine empathic summary.

6. Basic role plays take 3–5 min; more complex interviews, such as family interviews, usually take 7–10 min—sometimes up to 20 min.

7. "Mistakes" are accepted as part of the process of learning. They are opportunities, not catastrophes.

8. A trainee or faculty member can call for a time out whenever the interview seems to be stuck. A useful approach to a stuck interview can be to help the interviewer access what he or she is experiencing emotionally by asking: *What are you experiencing as you talk to this family?* A follow-up question: *What meaning does this have for you?* can help the trainee become aware of any internal block he or she has to being present and nonjudgmental with the patient.

9. Utilize reverse role play: a teacher demonstrates the skill to be learned. An interviewing technique is initially demonstrated to everyone in the group. Occasionally, the trainer will briefly demonstrate a technique during the middle of a role play when a student encounters a problematic interaction. The teacher models a willingness to be vulnerable by interviewing under the scrutiny of others [1].

10. Participants should stay in role most of the time, but times of laughter are inevitable and desirable [1]. One of the most powerful attributes of role-playing as a teaching tool is the fun participants can experience.

11. Externalize the thoughts of the interviewer [6]. For example, a resident appears anxious and stuck while assessing a suicidal adolescent. During a timeout in the interview, she worries that she may say the 'wrong thing.' Another resident then stands next to her as she tries to talk with the adolescent, whispering: *You may say the wrong thing.* The interviewer then experiences how hard it is to connect with a patient when she talks to herself like that.

12. Interviewing and relationship skills are essential components of being an effective clinician. Trainees are not asked to volunteer to participate in role plays any more than a surgical resident is asked to volunteer for a simulated gallbladder surgery exercise. Trainees are expected to participate. Otherwise, some trainees will avoid role-playing altogether. Most trainees respond to gentle encouragement: *Joe, why don't you be the doctor in this role play* [1]. In fact, the participants expect this, since it was agreed upon in the original contract. (A trainee with a phobia is the exception.)

13. An important goal of this text is to give trainees the literal words they might say. The interviewer is occasionally given an index card with specific questions or statements on them. A sample card, demonstrating the third-person technique, might say: *Lots of times, parents of babies who have cough and congestion worry about their breathing, that they might stop breathing. Is that true for you?* Over time, the trainee will transform the words into his or her own unique way of interviewing and relating.

Feedback to Trainees

Trainees want and need feedback on their progress. Almost every year at our annual first-year resident retreat, trainees request more frequent feedback on their performances. Without feedback, trainees are left with one of two conclusions: (1) faculty members are not interested, or (2) I must be doing it well since nobody is saying otherwise. Teachers of interviewing skills know the second conclusion is not warranted. It is not uncommon for a trainee to have good medical knowledge, present patients well, and in general appear competent, yet fall short when his or her interviewing skills are directly observed. Interviewing skills must be demonstrated in order to know a trainee is competent. A trainee can easily be unaware of nonverbal or other interviewing behaviors that are problematic [1].

A second principle underlying the feedback given in this text is rooted in the belief that people do best when they feel good about themselves and are excited about what they are learning. Consequently, feedback needs to be nonpersonal and balanced, with the positives outweighing the negatives. This allows the trainee to build on a positive base, and it encourages him or her to be responsible for learning the skills.

All feedback examples in this text are given within a small group context. The leader of the small group meets with the group members in a circle so everyone has eye contact with any other group members. The leader sees himself or herself as a facilitator, and does not monopolize the talking [7]. Since the group consists of four to six members, ample opportunity exists for students or residents to take turns role-playing. (Residents form groups with residents, students form groups with other students.) I have found that residents and students are willing to experiment with role plays in groups of this size.

Feedback to the Interviewer has the Following Characteristics:

1. Feedback is based on the mutual objectives discussed before the role play begins. Trainees can be asked what specific feedback they are looking for at the time the objectives are discussed. Ideally, the objectives for a specific role play fit in with the broader interviewing goals or contract with that trainee.
2. The group leader begins the feedback phase by asking the interviewer what he or she liked about his or her interview. The leader also asks for affirmations from others. The person playing the patient gives important information about what it felt like being the patient [6]. Affirmations are most effective when they note specific behaviors, perhaps exact quotes [7]. That means the mentor must take notes of specific statements made during the interview to be able to provide effective feedback. Affirmations do not need to be effusive to be effective. Occasionally, they are given in the middle of an interview to mark a desired behavioral technique [1]. Affirmations are stated to the interviewer directly: *I thought you made a good use of silence in the interview.* If participants talk about the interviewer, they are asked to speak directly to the interviewer. This encourages the interviewer to more fully absorb the affirmation. If the interviewer brushes the affirmation aside, the leader might respond: *Joe, did you take in the affirmation from Bill?*
3. Once all affirmations are given, the participants in the group are asked if they have any options. Sometimes, interviewers want to give themselves options before all the affirmations are given. It is best for them to wait, so that the affirmation phase is not shortchanged. Options are another way of doing the interview.

They are not meant to convey to the interviewer that he or she did it wrong. A good interview can be accomplished in a variety of ways. Even though options are not meant to be critical, it is possible that a trainee will interpret it that way. A leader can check this by routinely asking: *What is it like to get this feedback?* Any negative emotions can be acknowledged and processed. It is important to limit options to one or two key themes, so that the trainee does not feel overwhelmed.

4. Often the trainee is asked to repeat the exercise to demonstrate he or she has benefitted from the feedback and has really learned the skill. This is very important [6]. Typically, this leads to improvement, and allows the role play to end in a place of victory.

5. Feedback in long, complex interviews can also be given during the middle of the interview by signaling "time out" and providing corrective feedback. This allows the interviewer to make a quick adjustment [4].

6. Feedback that encourages trainees to internally reflect on their own thoughts and feelings as they interview is essential. Trainees often need to experience the warmth and consistency of the faculty mentor over time before they feel safe to acknowledge personal issues impacting the interview [1].

Self-Awareness

Staying self-aware is the process of developing, in the present moment, "insight into how one's life experiences and emotional make-up affect one's interactions with patients, families, and other professionals" [8]. It is essential to a patient-centered approach to interviewing. Self-awareness brings the process into the exam room. It is dynamic and immediate. Increased clinician self-awareness is associated with better patient outcomes, enhanced clinician satisfaction, and avoidance of burnout [9, 10]. These are no small advantages.

> One afternoon early in my career, in the middle of an influenza epidemic, I was behind schedule. I entered the room of an 8-year-old boy with cystic fibrosis, accompanied by his father. The father immediately greeted me with anger about his long wait. Reacting with no insight, I responded in kind, "I'm doing the best that I can. Lots of children are sick today." This reaction was fueled by my thoughts: I am usually on schedule, and I have gone out of my way for your child many times.

If I had stayed aware of my process, I would have noticed that I was rushed and feeling some pressure to see a number of patients in a limited time. I could have managed that anxiety, reminded myself that taking care of this patient in the past did not entitle me to be late, and simply apologized to this father for being late.

In addition to the immediate context of a clinician–patient interaction like the one above, trainees may experience relationships in practice that resemble relationships from their family of origin. These resemblances can trigger positive or negative interactions with patients and families, especially when the resemblances are unrecognized. Trainees take care of families with histories of trauma and emotional neglect, families grieving significant losses, as well as families dealing with a host of acute and chronic illnesses. These situations can be powerful triggers to trainees who had similar experiences in their own past. The feelings appear reflexively. If unrecognized, they determine the reaction of the clinician.

> A new trainee quickly picked up a caseload of families with complex and difficult psycho-social problems. She was the last one to finish with the patients in continuity clinic, often staying much later than her colleagues to finish her work. She felt a strong pull to help these multi-problem families. She was overwhelmed with the extent of their problems and their sense of helplessness. She worked harder and harder. She would give advice and recommendations for change. The families responded, predictably, with resistance. The resident felt depleted. She sought consultation from one of her mentors.

This resident acknowledged her pattern of attempting to rescue distressed families, overworking, and the inevitable emotional depletion that follows rescuing.[2] She did not recognize initially that her depleted state prevented her from fully joining and partnering with these families. This trainee traced the origin of her rescuing pattern to witnessing her brother suffer physically and psychologically with a childhood cancer. Once she recognized this connection to her past, she was in a position to change her pattern. Resemblances to current family situations act identically to family-of-origin connections [11]. For instance, a clinician who has a family member who recently experienced a delayed diagnosis of colon cancer may become overly forceful in recommending colonoscopy screening to his patients.

The ongoing role-playing group, led by a faculty member, provides a good avenue to recognize and talk about these types of problematic reactions [12]. He or she repeatedly invites trainees to stay self-aware when they appear stuck in a role play or do not appear to be tracking with what the patient is saying: *Tell me what you are feeling emotionally or What are you thinking as the patient says…?* An interviewer might then be asked if the situation is familiar or similar to a family-of-origin issue for him or her. This is done in the context of a clear contract. Recall, the members of the group have already agreed to a contract and confidentiality. Members of the group easily acknowledge emotions they are experiencing in the moment. They are then helped to see the impact of their emotions on the interview. Some are able to connect the feeling to a similar feeling experienced in their family of origin. These are not explored in depth, since this is not a therapy group [13].

> A resident was talking to parents of a child in the hospital, who had unexpected bad news learned from a recent imaging study. The mother was upset. Instead of supporting the mother's upset feelings, which was one of the main objectives of the role play, he was trying to talk her out of feeling upset and defending himself. A time out was taken and the resident was asked what he was experiencing. He acknowledged feeling guilty that the mother was feeling badly. He wanted to help her feel better. He connected his thoughts and feelings to learning to be a helper in his family-of-origin. He did not discuss this in depth, but was able to make a connection between his feelings and over controlling this interview. He did a second role play from a very different position. He was calm, emotionally present and empathic with the mother during the replay.

---

[2]Rescuing is a pattern of interacting commonly seen in alcoholic families.

Smith et al. point out other common feelings elicited during role play, such as fears of losing control, appearing unpleasant, harming the patient, and of being reminded of one's own personal issues, such as a difficult divorce [13]. These feelings can result in avoidance of psychological material, under control, and over control of the interview, as in the above scenario. Although simply identifying the response led to change with this resident, often the trainee changes only after repeated feedback [13].

Diagnostic Acumen

There is an additional, important advantage to staying self-aware and attending to the present moment. It enhances the data gathering function of the interview. A clinician who stays in the moment can be curious about missing or inconsistent data and not jump to conclusions.

> A preadolescent girl is rushed to the ER with respiratory distress. She has a history of asthma. She developed trouble breathing upon arrival at school—just an hour ago. She complained she couldn't catch her breath. Vital signs exam in the ER reveal tachycardia and tachypnea. She appears to be in marked distress, putting all her effort into each deep breath. On auscultation, she is moving air well and has inspiratory wheezing, most prominent in the upper airway. No expiratory prolongation or wheezing. Her oxygen saturation is 98 percent. The resident is anxious and quickly orders back-to-back albuterol nebulizer treatments, without any change occurring in her clinical status. His diagnosis: asthma. He consults with the ER attending who provides an alternative diagnosis: paradoxical vocal cord motion and anxiety. Improvement occurs once the anxiety is managed.

The resident developed anxious thoughts about this child's condition, imagined all kinds of bad outcomes, and acted on that anxiety. He did not stay curious and in the moment, so he missed the fact that the child had sudden onset of respiratory distress, unlike her usual asthma presentation. In addition, the resident discounted physical exam findings of stridor and good air entry, as well as an oxygen saturation of 98 percent. If this resident had allowed himself to stay aware, to be curious about these findings, he might have considered alternative diagnoses.

Key Points

1. Trainee anxiety is the chief barrier to role plays.
2. Role play has many advantages for teaching interviewing skills to trainees.
3. Faculty members establish safety in the role-playing group by joining with the trainees, contracting, expressing empathy, and giving affirmations freely.
4. Trainees, like the rest of humanity, have a natural drive to protect themselves from feeling the pain associated with vulnerable feelings.
5. Trainees may have had little experience in recognizing their own feelings.

6. Self-awareness is essential to good patient care.
7. Talking to peers and faculty in a group setting can help physicians stay aware of family-of-origin influences that might adversely affect patient care.
8. Staying curious and in the moment can help a clinician avoid jumping to conclusions about the diagnosis.
9. Go slowly. Let the trainees be the guide.

Teaching to Use Role-Play Transcripts

A faculty mentor has a variety of options for teaching with the cases found at the beginning of Chap. 1–20, exclusive of 12. He or she can utilize the brief case description with suggested objectives as the basis for a spontaneous role play by the trainee and patient actor. If only the objectives from the case are used, the trainee can present a case from his or her own practice, which might enhance the trainee's investment in the role play. The faculty member might also present a de novo case to teach an interviewing technique not covered in the role-play examples. For instance, he or she may use a guiding technique to help a patient adopt a healthier eating pattern. Even though the actual scripts are not likely to be read aloud or acted out, they do provide concrete examples of using role play to teach interviewing skills.

References

1. Barney C, Shea SC. The art of effectively teaching clinical interviewing skills using role-playing: a primer. Psychiatr Clin North Am. 2007;30:e31–50.
2. Baker S, Daniels T. Integrating research on the microcounseling program: a meta-analysis. J Couns Psychol. 1989;36:213–22.
3. Crabb W, Moracco J, Bender R. A comparative study of empathy training with program instruction for lay helpers. J Couns Psychol. 1983;30:221–6.
4. Shea SC, Barney C. Macrotraining: A "how-to" primer for using serial role-playing to train complex clinical interviewing tasks such as suicide assessment. Psychiatr Clin North Am. 2007;30:e1–29.
5. Shea SC. Psychiatric interviewing: the art of understanding: a practical guide for psychiatrists, psychologists, counselors, social workers, nurses, and other mental health professionals. 2nd ed. Philadelphia, PA: WB Saunders; 1998.
6. Cole SA, Bird J, Monce R. Teaching with role-play: a structured approach. In: Lipkin M, Putnam SM, Lazare A, editors. The medical interview: clinical care, education, and research. New York, NY: Springer; 1995.
7. Turner TL, Palazzi DL, Ward MA. The clinical-educator's handbook. Houston: Baylor College of Medicine; 2008.
8. Novack DH, Suchman AL, Clark W, Epstein RM, Najberg E, Kaplan C, et al. Calibrating the physician: personal awareness and effective patient care. JAMA. 1997;278:502–9.
9. Epstein R. Mindful practice in action (1); technical competence, evidence-based medicine, and relationship-centered care. Fam Syst Health. 2003;21:1–19.

10. Suchman AL, Roter D, Green M, Lipkin M, The Collaborative Study Group of the American Academy on Physician and Patient. Physician satisfaction with primary care office visits. Med Care. 1993;31:1083–92.
11. McDaniel SH, Campbell TL, Hepworth S, Lorenz A. Chapter 26 – Managing personal and professional boundaries: how the clinician's own experience can be a resource in patient care. In: McDaniel SH, Campbell TL, Hepworth S, Lorenz A, editors. Family-oriented primary care. 2nd ed. New York, NY: Springer; 2005. p. 450–64.
12. McDaniel SH, Campbell TL, Mancini J, Shore B. Using a group as a consultant. In: Wynne L, McDaniel SH, Weber T, editors. System consultation: a new perspective for family therapy. New York, NY: Guilford Press; 1986.
13. Smith RC, Dwamena FC, Fortin AH. Teaching personal awareness. J Gen Intern Med. 2005;20:201–7.

Chapter 1
Personal Story

"The good physician treats the disease.
The great physician treats the patient who has the disease."

William Osler

Role Play

Prerequisite interviewing skills for role playing the personal story include *gentle commands, facilitation or continuers, listening, and tracking*. (See glossary for a description of terms.)

Role Play: A 26-year-old mother brings her 5-day-old baby for her first checkup. The pregnancy and delivery were uneventful. The baby is a little fussy, but otherwise doing well.

Objectives

1. Obtain the personal story.
2. Persist in getting the story.

Clinician	Ms. Green, I'm Dr. Murphy, one of the pediatric residents.
Patient	Hello.
Clinician	Before I ask you questions and check your baby, I would like you to tell me about yourself.
Patient	What do you mean?
Clinician	I would like you to tell me about yourself personally.
Patient	I'm 26.
Clinician	Please go on.

(continued)

The online version of this chapter (doi:10.1007/978-1-4614-7224-7_5) contains supplementary material, which is available to authorized users.

Patient	Sarah is my first baby. Right now I'm living with my parents. I'm single.
Clinician	Tell me more about yourself.
Patient	I'm excited about Sarah—not so much about living with my parents.
Clinician	Say more.
Patient	I'm worried about living with my parents. My mom and I have not gotten along well in the past.
Clinician	You have not gotten along well with your mother, and you are worried about how it will work for you and your baby?
Patient	That's right.
Clinician	What's it been like for you so far?
Patient	Not good. I'm uptight. The baby is fussy.
Clinician	The baby is fussy?
Patient	I don't know if she has too much gas.
Clinician	So, you are concerned that the fussiness could possibly be due to the gas?

Feedback

Faculty	Okay, let's stop. (*to trainee*) Tell me what you did well in the interview.
Trainee	I'm not sure.
Patient	Well, I thought you showed interest in me. You made good eye contact and invited me to talk. You listened well. You were nonjudgmental.
Trainee	What do I need to improve?
Faculty	Did you take in that affirmation?
Trainee	Probably not.
Faculty	You might consider taking in the affirmation and letting yourself feel good about what you are already doing. I thought you did a strong interview. You gave the patient plenty of space to talk. You had a warm manner, and you persisted in getting the personal story with open-ended inquiries. You did not try to focus her on one topic. You let her talk about what she thought was important, and she did.
Trainee	Thanks.

(continued)

Faculty	Would you like to hear options now? Remember, options are not meant to be criticisms—they are just another way of conducting the interview. There is no one 'right way' to do the interview.
Trainee	Yes.
Patient	I thought asking me about my personal story seemed a little abrupt. A short explanation after I asked, "What do you mean?" might help.
Trainee	It did feel awkward to me, too.
Faculty	I have an introduction that you might try… Tell the patient why you are asking for personal information. Once patients understand the rationale, they usually are happy to share their story with you. I wrote the introduction down on an index card. I suggest you replay from the beginning of the interview, using this introduction. Stay aware of any difference you notice between the two interviews.
Trainee	Okay.

Replay

Trainee	Hello, Ms. Green. I'm Doctor Murphy, a pediatric resident.
Patient	Hello.
Trainee	(*reading from the index card*) I'll be asking you questions and checking your baby in a few minutes. I find it helpful to get to know people personally before asking about medical stuff. I believe I can give better care when I know who and what are important in the person's life. Would you be willing to start by telling me about yourself?
Patient	Sure. I'm 26 years old and Sarah is my first child. I am a single mother, currently living with my parents. I am not excited about that, but I am very excited about Sarah. I love her to death. She's even better than I imagined.
Trainee	It sounds like you really enjoy your baby.
Patient	I do. But sometimes it is hard to have time with just her. My family can be over involved.
Trainee	Uh-huh.
Patient	Sometimes I just want to have the baby totally to myself. I know my mother just wants to be helpful. However, she can be annoying.

Feedback

Faculty	Okay, let's stop. (*to trainee*) Did this interview feel any different than the first one?
Trainee	It felt more natural and smooth.
Patient	It did not seem abrupt at all.
Faculty	Why was that?
Patient	I understood why the physician was asking me about myself. I wanted to tell him the second time.
Faculty	Good.

Obstacles to Teaching Personal Story

1. Medical training, in general, is based on a biomedical model.
2. Interviewer is anxious about asking for psychosocial information.
3. Interviewer is concerned that obtaining the personal story will take too much time.

Strategies

1. Teach trainees about the strong scientific evidence supporting a biopsychosocial approach.
2. Demonstrate how to obtain the personal story. Model it in day-to-day practice.
3. Teach structure techniques so trainees develop confidence in guiding the interview (see chapter 7).

Personal Story

William Hurt, playing an attending physician in the movie, *The Doctor*, berates a surgical resident after the resident identified a patient as "the terminal" during hospital rounds. It is a dramatic and poignant moment in the movie. That resident missed the person of the patient—just as we do when we label a patient as 'a leukemic', 'a diabetic', or 'a borderline.' Due to his own struggle with laryngeal cancer, William Hurt had discovered the importance of viewing patients as people in the context of their personal story, family relationships, hopes and dreams. However, he had not yet learned the importance of also treating trainees in this manner. Sadly, it can take a major loss, such as what William Hurt's character experienced, before one can truly appreciate the importance of knowing patients as people.

Knowing and connecting with the person in the patient deepens engagement and provides an environment in which patients feel free to openly communicate [1]. Satisfaction of both the clinician and the patient are clearly enhanced [1, 2]. The history is more complete and accurate, and there is improvement in the outcome [2–4].

Clinicians in primary care often generate extensive differential diagnoses, even when patients present with common symptoms. Diagnostic lists, mostly made up of physical conditions, can lead to costly workups [5]. As much as 75 percent of the time, the workup is negative [6]. Psychosocial conditions, such as depression, anxiety, stress, and somatoform disorders all can present with physical symptoms—many go undiagnosed and untreated [7–9]. A biopsychosocial approach addresses these problems by integrating the physical with the emotional or psychological data from the very beginning [10]. The biopsychosocial interview starts with the personal story [10, 11].

Clinician	I am interested in getting to know you as a person before we start talking about your concerns. Tell me about yourself, personally.
Patient	I'm 26 years old. I work....

The vast majority of patients are happy to tell the clinician their stories in 1–2 minutes. Occasional patients may appear reluctant and respond with a statement like: *What do you want to know?* A simple reply often stimulates the patient to talk: *Whatever you think is most important* [11]. Alternatively, the underlying rationale can be fully explained:

"I think my job is to understand as much as I can about you and about the troubles you're having. It helps me to help you if I know who you are, what your life is about, and who is in your life." [11, p. 45]

Once patients begin to tell their stories, open-ended inquiries encourage them to expand their stories without premature focusing on details.

Patient	I really enjoy taking care of my children, but it can be hard to balance home and work.
Clinician	Tell me more.
Patient	My boss gets on my case and makes me feel guilty whenever I have to take time off to take care of a sick child. I think the stress is affecting my health.

Sometimes the personal story will be directly related to the symptoms. Even when this is not the case, the patient will be placing his or her symptoms in context, allowing the physician to appreciate his or her illness (as opposed to disease).

It is important to stay aware that the personal story differs from the small talk that can accompany clinicians' visits. Small talk, such as discussion of sporting events or the local weather, does not lead to a better understanding of the patient as a person [11].

If the personal story is not obtained at the beginning of the interview due to the acuity of the patient's symptoms (e.g., acute pain, respiratory distress) or for any other reason, a clinician may be able to obtain that data later [11].

Clinician	I feel I have a good understanding of your abdominal pain. I would like to take a step back for a second and find out about you as a person. It helps me give better care when I understand the bigger picture. Tell me about yourself, personally.
Patient	Okay, I'm....

Key Points

1. The personal story is fundamental to a biopsychosocial approach.
2. The personal story takes 1–2 min to obtain.
3. Curiosity and learning about patients as people greatly increase clinician satisfaction with medical practice.
4. Any clinician can learn to obtain the personal story.
5. Obtaining the personal story enhances both engagement and open-ended inquiry with patients.

References

1. Platt FW, Garspar DL, Coulehan JL, Fox L, Adler AJ, Weston WW, et al. "Tell me about yourself": the patient-centered interview. Ann Intern Med. 2001;134:1079–85.
2. Safran DG, Taira DA, Rogers WH, Kosinski M, Ware JE, Tarlov AR. Linking primary care performance to outcomes of care. J Fam Pract. 1998;47:213–20.
3. Linfors EW, Neelon FA. Interrogation and interview: strategies for obtaining clinical data. J R Coll Gen Practit. 1981;31:426–8.
4. Kaplan SH, Greenfield S, Ware JE. Assessing the effects of physician-patient interactions on the outcomes of chronic disease. Med Care. 1989;27:s110–23.
5. Kroenke K, Price RK. Symptoms in the community: prevalence, classification, and psychiatric comorbidity. Arch Intern Med. 1993;153:2474–80.

6. Kroenke K, Mangelsdorff D. Common symptoms in ambulatory care: incidence, evaluation, therapy, and outcome. Am J Med. 1989;86:262–6.

7. Deacon B, Lickel J, Abromwitz JS. Medical utilization across the anxiety disorders. J Anxiety Disord. 2008;22:344–50.

8. Sartorius N, Ustun TB, Lecrubier Y, Wittehen H-U. Depression comorbid with anxiety: results from the WHO study on psychological disorders in primary health care. Br J Psychiatry. 1996;168 Suppl 30:38–43.

9. Platt FW, McMath JC. Clinical hypocompetence: the interview. Ann Intern Med. 1979;91: 898–902.

10. Fortin A, Dwamena FC, Frankel RM, Smith RC. Smith's patient-centered interviewing: an evidence-based method. 3rd ed. New York, NY: McGraw Hill; 2012.

11. Platt FW, Gordon GH. Field guide to the difficult patient interview. 2nd ed. Philadelphia, PA: Lippincott William and Wilkins; 2004.

Chapter 2
Contracting

Role Play

Pre-requisite interviewing skills for role-playing contracting with a patient include *open-ended inquiries, listening, and tracking*.

Role Play #1: A 57-year-old woman, scheduled for a 20-minute follow up visit, presents with a list of the following items: back and joint pains, tiredness, heartburn, occasional urinary incontinence, anxiety, and insomnia.

Objective

Establish a clear contract for the visit.

Trainee	Hi, Mrs. Gordon. I'm glad you made a list. Tell me what is most important that we deal with today, from your standpoint.
Patient	My difficulty sleeping is my biggest problem right now.
Trainee	We will evaluate that. I think it would be important to check out your tiredness since that is a new symptom. It's possible that one or two of the other problems are related to that.
Patient	It's possible.
Trainee	I don't think there is time to adequately evaluate all the other symptoms today. Why don't we schedule a follow up for those?
Patient	Okay.

The online version of this chapter (doi:10.1007/978-1-4614-7224-7_5) contains supplementary material, which is available to authorized users.

J. Binder, *Primary Care Interviewing: Learning Through Role Play*,
DOI 10.1007/978-1-4614-7224-7_2, © Springer Science+Business Media New York 2013

Feedback

Faculty	Let's stop. (*to trainee*) What did you like about your interview?
Trainee	I felt comfortable negotiating with the patient.
Faculty	(*to patient*) What did you like about the interview?
Actor	I felt you (*trainee*) were considerate of my needs. Setting an agenda for the visit made sense to me.
Faculty	I agree with the above. When you set limits for the visit, you are more likely to feel calm and not rushed. Anybody else have affirmations?
Trainee #2	I thought the interview was efficient and smooth. I like the way you affirmed her for bringing the list.
Faculty	Anybody have options?
Group	(*no response*)
Faculty	Okay. Good job.

Role Play #2:   A 7-year-old girl has had recurrent abdominal pain for 6 weeks. This is her initial evaluation for abdominal pain.

Objective

Establish a contract with the family to inquire about both biomedical and psychosocial factors that may be contributing to her pain.

Trainee	Anna, would you like to color some pictures while I start off asking your mother and father some questions?
Child	Sure.
Trainee	Mr. & Mrs. Long, I would like to hear from each of you regarding the main reason for the visit today.
Mother	Anna has abdominal pain. I would like to find out what is causing it—to make sure it is nothing serious. Anna seems okay when she doesn't have the pain. She plays normally. She is not running any fevers. To tell you the truth, I'm a bit perplexed. That is why we didn't bring her in right away. She has not had any vomiting or diarrhea.
Trainee	Does she show you where her belly hurts?

(continued)

Mother	She points to her belly button.
Trainee	Has she had any change in her appetite or weight loss?
Mother	None. She always has been a picky eater.
Trainee	Does she have trouble tolerating particular foods?
Mother	Not really.
Trainee	How about any urinary symptoms?
Mother	No.
Trainee	Okay. Mr. Long, what concerns do you have?
Mother	I have had the same concerns as my wife.
Trainee	So you both want to figure out the cause of the pain to make sure it is not serious?
Parents	Yes.
Trainee	Let me tell you, first off, that abdominal pain in children has lots of causes. It can be due to problems in the bowels, infections or even stresses that children face nowadays. Is it okay if I ask you about all that?
Parents	Sure.

Feedback

Faculty	(*to trainee*) What do you think you did well?
Trainee	I think I explained what I was going to do, and I got their agreement to a contract for the session.
Faculty	Yes. You got their agreement to discuss biomedical and psychosocial factors.
Trainee 2	I thought having Anna color while you talked with the parents was an excellent idea.
Faculty	I also liked the way you asked each parent about their main reason for the visit. Does anybody have options?
Group	(*no response*)
Faculty	I have one option. The mother began to give the history of present illness before the father expressed his hopes for the session. I suggest getting that agreement before moving to the history of present illness.
Trainee	That makes sense.
Faculty	Let's run through it one more time.

Replay

Trainee	Anna, would you like to color pictures, while I ask your mother and father some questions?
Child	Yes.
Trainee	Mr. & Mrs. Long, I would like to hear from each of you regarding the main reason for the visit today.
Mother	Anna has had abdominal pain off and on for 6 weeks. I am starting to grow concerned about her, and want to make sure it is not something serious. She plays just like usual. She doesn't have vomiting or diarrhea.
Trainee	Mrs. Long, would it be okay if I came back to the history in one minute. I would like to talk for a minute all together about what we are going to do during today's visit, to make sure we get everything accomplished. Is that okay?
Mother	Sure.
Trainee	Mr. Long, let me hear from you about your major concern or reason for the visit.
Father	It really is the same as my wife's.
Trainee	So, you both want to understand the cause of the pain and make sure it is nothing serious. Abdominal pain in children can be due to a number of different conditions.

Feedback

Faculty	Let me jump in here. You did a nice job of stopping mom from moving to the history of present illness without being abrasive. You stayed in the region of contracting with the family. Good job.

Obstacles to Teaching Contracting

1. Interviewer holds an old-school paternalistic approach to patients, one in which the doctor directs the interaction.
2. Interviewer does not have the specific word skills to establish a clear contract.

3. Trainee does not understand contract renegotiation may be necessary as more information becomes available.
4. Interviewer fears that he or she will not be able to fulfill an explicit agreement made with a patient.

Strategies

1. Educate trainees about the empirical evidence showing collaboration leads to better health outcomes.
2. Initially, give the interviewer the words to say to the patient, until he or she develops his or her own unique style.
3. Educate trainees about the importance of the initial contract and reevaluating the initial contract, especially if the clinician-patient interaction is stuck.
4. Help trainees learn that contracts hold both patients and clinicians accountable for their actions. Fulfilling contracts helps to build trust.

Contracting

The empirical evidence is robust: partnership improves health outcomes [1, 2]. Both the patient and clinician report more satisfaction when they perceive the relationship as a partnership [1]. Agreement on a clear contract is necessary for an effective partnership. A contract is "an explicit bilateral commitment to a well-defined course of action" [3]. An agenda is established for each visit and role responsibilities for each partner in the long-term relationship are clarified. Unrealistic expectations are avoided. Both the clinician and patient have a framework for discussing medical problems and unhealthy lifestyle behaviors—such as smoking and poor nutrition—in a collaborative manner, not an adversarial one. Solid contracts instill hope [4].

Effective contracts are:

1. **Specific and clear**. *Doctor, I am having shoulder pain. I want to find out what is causing the pain and get some relief.* This patient and doctor have a map for what will likely happen during the visit. Of course, contracting in primary care practice often is not so simple. Adult patients typically present with more than one problem [5, 6]. The clinician and patient must prioritize the list and negotiate an acceptable agenda for the visit. Some problems, especially those regarding emotional or psychosocial issues, may not even be mentioned initially [7, 8].

The following dialogue during the opening phase of a checkup for a 50-year-old woman with diabetes and shoulder pain, is simple and clear.

Patient	My shoulder has been bothering me.
Clinician	Let's set an agenda for the visit today. Do you want to put that as one of the items on your list?
Patient	Yes. My shoulder has really been painful.
Clinician	Anything else?
Patient	No.
Clinician	I would like to check on your diabetes as well.
Patient	Okay.

The clinician and the patient in the above case quickly agree on their expectations for their time together. Sometimes, patients start telling details of the present illness, as in the second role play above, before an agreement for the agenda has been reached. If the clinician does not interrupt that process and finalize the contract, the goals of the patient and clinician for the visit may remain unclear and unmet.

Clinician	**What are your hopes for our time together**?
Patient	My shoulder has been bothering me.
Clinician	Let's set an agenda for the visit today. Do you want to put that as one of the items on our list?
Patient	Yes. My shoulder has really affected me. I can't get any relief. The pain is shooting down my arm. The worst part is my sleep. I may sleep for 2–3 hours, and then I'm awake again. I have to get some relief.
Clinician	That sounds very difficult. Before we discuss your shoulder, I would like to make sure we have our agenda set for our time together. I would like to check on your diabetes, as well.
Patient	That sounds fine.
Clinician	Anything else?
Patient	No.

Specific contracts call for accountability from the patient and the clinician to act in ways to fulfill the contract. Negotiating a clear contract for the not only the visit, but also the overall nature of the relationship, helps avoid surprises and encourages cooperation. An example of such a detailed contract for routine care might go like this:

Clinician	I would like to talk with you about how I see our relationship over time. I believe that my job as a doctor is to provide the best comprehensive care that I can. That means taking care of you when you have the flu or a chronic illness, like diabetes. In addition, since emotional health and physical health are parts of one whole, I will ask you how you are doing emotionally from time to time. And, I will need to ask you about high risk health behaviors, such as smoking. Is that okay with you?
Patient	I expect no less from you.

Eric Berne emphasized the importance of clarity in contracting with a story he told at his last public lecture in 1970. "I once got on an airplane and the pilot came over the loudspeaker and said, 'This flight is going toward New York.' I said, 'Let me out. I want to go to New York.'" [9]

Psychosocial Issues

The increased effort commonly involved in obtaining clarity with a psychosocial issue makes it tempting for the clinician to settle for a vague contract. It is important for the clinician to avoid that temptation, because vague contracts lead to futility. Since emotional factors can act as a barrier to the establishment of a good contract, eliciting the patient's feelings, clarifying the issue, and educating the patient are essential preliminary tasks. (See Chaps. 14 and 18 for further development of contracting with psychosocial issues.)

A 60-year-old man, who has had insulin dependent diabetes mellitus for a decade, presents to the clinic. He has lost a fair amount of vision secondary to retinal changes. He has been sporadically monitoring his blood sugars and diet. He has not attended regular medical visits with his primary care physician. The patient says he wants to take good care of his diabetes and prevent further vision loss. He has not been adherent to standard treatment recommendations in the past secondary to his fear. He does not check his blood sugars, so he won't see a high number. He has been avoiding the physician in order not to hear bad news. The clinician elicits all this information through gentle inquiry and then helps him with his feelings and distorted thinking. Only then is the patient in a position to commit to a healthy contract.

CONTRACT: I will resolve my fear of hearing bad news about my diabetes. I will attend my regularly scheduled visits to monitor my diabetes. I will monitor my glucose levels and diet as recommended. My goal is to improve my vision.

Patient fear was an obstacle to providing good clinical care in the above case. It highlights the importance of understanding a patient's cognitive framework and associated feelings before contracting on psychosocial issues. The following inquiry is a helpful way to introduce the topic: *What has it been like for you to live with a chronic condition like diabetes?*

2. **Positively stated**. The absence of a behavior is hard to visualize. A person visualizing 'not smoking' will automatically picture the act of smoking. A positively worded contract gives the patient a direction and a course of action to take instead of smoking. This can be effective in and of itself [10]. Perhaps, a patient agrees to: *I will take a walk or talk to my wife whenever I feel an urge to smoke.*
3. **Renegotiable.** Patients must specify what they are hoping for, as a result of the visit, or a result of the ongoing clinician-patient relationship. However, as we have just noted, many patients do not reveal their primary concern initially. In addition, as the clinician learns more about who his or her patient is and what is important to this patient, the clinician will be better able help the patient create a more focused contract—one attuned to the patient's needs.

Clinician	Some of my other patients with diabetes have told me that they sometimes avoid checking their glucose level because they don't want to see a high result and then feel discouraged. Does that ever happen with you?
Patient	I have to admit that is true.
Clinician	Tell me what you feel emotionally at that time?
Patient	If I have not been eating well, I do fear checking my glucose. So, I might not check and just hope it is okay.
Clinician	That sounds like a difficult situation. I know you want to protect your eyesight and stay out of the hospital. It might be worthwhile for us to talk about your fear and ways of managing it today. What do you think?
Patient	If you think it will help.

This patient experienced empathy from the clinician and was then willing to re-focus the contract. This is an important principle: **contact before contract**, especially when contracting for any lifestyle or behavioral change [11].

Mini contracts

Clinicians can support the process of partnering with their patients by asking permission to ask further questions. In a way, they are simply solidifying the initial contract. This can be especially effective when giving a treatment recommendation or discussing a sensitive topic [12].

Clinician	May I ask you a few more questions about what has made it so difficult to check your glucose level regularly?
Patient	Sure.

4. **Realistic, identifying achievable goals**. Both the clinician and patient have responsibilities here. The clinician must not agree to a list of actions which he or she cannot possibly accomplish. It is not realistic to diagnose and treat multiple somatic complaints, provide anticipatory guidance, and partner with the patient on a major lifestyle change—like smoking cessation—all within 20 minutes, just because they are listed on a computer form. Some clinicians attempt to deal with this time crunch by controlling the interview with closed-end questions, resulting in brief answers and a dissatisfied doctor and patient [5]. A better approach is to be realistic about what can be accomplished in 20 minutes and agree to a reasonable agenda: *So today, we will see how you are managing your diabetes and evaluate your shoulder pain. Do you agree to come back for a full check up in the next month or two, when we will evaluate what preventive health care you might need?*

Patient agreement to a contract must be realistic, as well. A patient, because of current life difficulties, might not be willing to do a specific treatment or make a lifestyle change. Or, the patient might not believe in his or her ability to perform some action or make a change. It is important for the patient not to be persuaded to agree to a contract that is not realistic for him or her right now. These issues must be resolved before a valid contract can be established. This might take multiple visits over months or even years.

Concrete examples of effective contracts are given throughout this text: with families, adolescents, somatically fixated patients, during wandering and shutdown interviews, sensitive interviews, as well as when dealing with patients considering making lifestyle or behavioral changes. These examples are intended to highlight one of the fundamental principles of clinician-patient relationships: **clear contracting is essential for effective partnership in any type of interview**. Occasionally, a clinician and patient may be unable to come to an agreement about a diagnostic workup or treatment plan. (Differences of opinion between the clinician and patient are covered in Chap. 20, as one of the examples of a challenging interview.)

One final note

The ability to contract is basic to successfully interviewing families and performing the more complex interviews in the second half of the book. A trainee who is having difficulty structuring a family interview or partnering with a patient or family often needs a brief refresher exercise on contracting. It is a common problem. A clear contract sets the structure for what is discussed during the middle and concluding phases of a family interview.

Key Points

1. Contracting supports a partnership.
2. Clear contracting leads to improved health outcomes [2].
3. Omission of contracting early in the interview can lead to becoming stuck later.
4. Contact before contract (even in busy primary care practices).
5. Contracting is a process. Renegotiate the contract when new information does not fit with the initial contract.
6. Contracting takes on increased importance with family interviews, as well as with complex or challenging interviews, such as a sensitive inquiry.

References

1. Stewart M, Brown JB, Weston WW. Patient-centered interviewing part III: five provocative questions. Can Fam Physician. 1989;35:159–61.
2. Starfield B, Wray C, Hess K, Gross R, Birk PS, D'Lugoff BC. The influence of patient-practitioner agreement on outcomes of care. Am J Public Health. 1981;71:127–32.
3. Joines V, Stewart I. TA today: a new introduction to transactional analysis. Chapel Hill, NC: Lifespace Publishing; 1987.
4. Baird JL. Contracting for change. In: Lenox CE, editor. Redecision therapy: a brief, action-oriented approach. Northvale, NJ: Jason Aronson Inc.; 1997.
5. Platt FW, Gordon GH. Field guide to the difficult patient interview. 2nd ed. Philadelphia, PA: Lippincott Williams and Wilkins; 2004.
6. Beckman HB, Frankel RM. The effect of physician behavior on the collection of data. Ann Intern Med. 1984;101:692–6.
7. Girón M, Majón-Arce P, Puerto-Barber J, Sánchez-Garcia E, Gómez-Beneyto M. Clinical interviewing skills and identification of emotional disorders in primary care. Am J Psychiatry. 1998;155:530–5.
8. White J, Levinson W, Roter D. "Oh by the way…": the closing moments of the medical visit. J Gen Intern Med. 1994;9:24–8.
9. Berne E. Away from a theory of the impact of interpersonal interaction on non-verbal participation. Transactional Anal J. 1971;1:6–13.
10. Stewart I. Transactional analysis counseling in action. 3rd ed. Los Angeles, CA: Sage; 2007.
11. Widdowson M. Transactional analysis: 100 key points and techniques. New York, NY: Routledge; 2010.
12. Epstein RM, Morse DS, Frankel RM, Frarey L, Anderson K, Beckman HB. Awkward moments in patient-physician communication about HIV risk. Ann Intern Med. 1998;128:435–47.

Chapter 3
Open-Ended Inquiry

Role Play

Prerequisite interviewing skills for role-playing open-ended inquiry include *gentle commands, facilitations, listening, empathic summaries*, and *tracking*.

Role Play #1: A 38-year-old woman, a new patient to the practice, presents with a history of fatigue and generalized musculoskeletal pains. She dates the onset to a car accident three years ago. She is telling the clinician her illness story.

Objectives

1. Use nonverbal techniques to create safety.
2. Demonstrate use of open-ended verbal techniques (facilitation, summarization, gentle commands, and open-ended questions) to encourage her to tell her story.

Trainee	Mrs. Bowen, tell me about the fatigue, the pains, and anything else you have experienced. Start at the beginning and walk me through the illness.
Patient	It began with my car accident 3 years ago. I had pain in my back and also my right shoulder and both legs after I got out of the hospital. Initially, I thought they would go away, but they didn't.

(continued)

J. Binder, *Primary Care Interviewing: Learning Through Role Play*,
DOI 10.1007/978-1-4614-7224-7_3, © Springer Science+Business Media New York 2013

Trainee	Okay.
Patient	In fact, the pains have worsened over time. I have been to a number of different doctors, physical therapists, pain specialists. I have received injections in my back, but they didn't help. Now, I can't even get my household chores done. I need help taking care of my children.
Trainee	Okay.
Patient	My husband has had to change his work schedule. I'm very dependent on him.
Trainee	Okay.
Patient	I'm very weak. My muscles feel like jelly.
Trainee	Tell me more about that.
Patient	My muscles just seem to have stopped working. I know it is not in my head. Nobody can tell me why.
Trainee	What do you think is the cause, even if you don't know for sure?
Patient	I think I probably injured something in my spine with the accident.
Trainee	Okay.

Feedback

Faculty	Let's stop. How about affirmations? (*to patient*) As the patient, what did you like about the interview?
Patient	I liked the way you (*trainee*) were interested in me. You made good eye contact and stayed quiet as you listened to my story.
Trainee #2	You used gentle commands and open-ended questions to encourage her to talk, such as, "Tell me more about that."
Trainee #3	I thought it was important that you asked her about her idea of why she was having symptoms.
Faculty	In addition, you listened without interrupting. You did not limit her by asking any closed-ended questions. Good job! Anybody have options?
Group	(*no response*)
Faculty	I have one option. That is your use of "okay" as a facilitating response. Sometimes it acts as a block to communication, especially when a patient is providing information that is not okay [1]. Platt and Gordon discuss the overuse of "okay" in their book, Field Guide to the Difficult Patient Interview. They suggest strategies for breaking the habit. Would you be willing to read about it and lead a brief discussion next week in our group meeting?
Trainee	Sure.

Role Play #2: A 54-year-old male has hypertension that has not responded to lifestyle changes. The clinician is recommending treatment with a diuretic.

Objectives

1. Recognize nonverbal signals of disengagement.
2. Use direct inquiry to address incongruence.

Trainee	Mr. Heinz, I would like to talk about your hypertension. You have done a good job of changing your diet and losing weight, but your blood pressure is still high.
Patient	I know.
Trainee	Given the level of your blood pressure, the standard recommendation is to start you on a diuretic.
Patient	(*Turns head away, averts eyes, and becomes silent.*)
Trainee	Mr. Heinz, hypertension can lead to all kinds of problems, including strokes. Diuretics have empirical evidence of effectiveness. I think it would help you to take a diuretic.
Patient	You are probably correct.

Feedback

Faculty	Okay, let's stop here. (*to trainee*) Tell me what you did well.
Trainee	I affirmed him for his weight loss. I thought I made good eye contact and went at a slow pace.
Faculty	I agree. You have a very warm, caring presence with patients. In this instance, your caring may have gotten in the way of recognizing and discussing his nonverbal signals of disengagement.
Trainee	I did notice he looked away. I wanted him to understand why he needs to take the diuretic.
Faculty	Taking the diuretic is important. However, until you understand and acknowledge his position, he is unlikely to hear your perspective. You might say something like the following statement as a way to open up the discussion, "I couldn't help notice you seemed to be a little hesitant when I mentioned medication. Do you have concerns?"
Trainee	I could do that.

Replay

Trainee	Mr. Heinz, I would like to talk about your hypertension. You have made wonderful changes with your weight. Only, it doesn't seem to be enough. The standard recommendation in your type of situation is to start medication.
Patient	(*Turns head away, averts eyes, and becomes silent.*)
Trainee	Mr. Heinz, the medication is safe and it works well.
Patient	Maybe.
Trainee	It's important that we not ignore your hypertension. We can prevent long-term problems.
Faculty	Okay, let's stop for now. (*to trainee*) How do you think it went?
Trainee	About the same. It is hard when the patient won't do what is best.
Faculty	It sure is. Why don't we come back to this again next week? Tell me what is like for you when patients don't follow our best advice?
Trainee	I get frustrated…
Faculty	Say more about that.
Trainee	I believe patients should take our recommendations for treatment, especially when the empirical evidence is solidly on our side.
Faculty	It sounds like you get very frustrated with patients who are nonadherent to our best recommendations.
Trainee	I do. I have spent a lot of time and effort learning medicine.
Faculty	I know you have worked hard. It has to be disappointing to see patients not take advantage of your knowledge.
Trainee	I guess I will have to learn to deal with it. It happens a lot.
Faculty	Yes it does.

Obstacles to Teaching Open-Ended Inquiry

1. Interviewer adopts a closed-ended questioning style after making one or two open-ended inquiries to initiate the interview.
2. Interviewer believes that patients will perceive empathic summaries as unnatural or condescending [2].

Strategies

1. Demonstrate the integration of open-ended and focused questioning with role reversal.
2. Give feedback to residents who quickly resort to a closed-ended questioning style.

3. Invite trainees to experiment with empathic summaries. They will likely discover that patients like them.
4. Suggest trainees introduce summaries with a statement, such as: *I'd like to check to see if I am hearing it correctly as we go along. Is that okay?* [1]

Open-Ended Inquiry

Careful analysis of hundreds of interviews in multiple scientific studies has demonstrated that a combination of open-ended inquiry and focused questioning to clarify details leads to the most complete database [3, 4, 5]. The common strategy of resorting to a series of closed-ended questions to save time is not supported by empirical evidence [5, 6]. Open-ended inquiry has an important additional benefit. Patients achieve better health outcomes when they are able to tell their story [7, 8]. Consequently, it is important for patients to feel free to tell their stories.

Create a Safe Environment

Patients open up and talk freely when they feel emotionally safe. A patient's level of feeling emotional safe is determined by his or her personality, as well as certain key characteristics of the clinician. A clinician creates a safe environment with an accepting, nonjudgmental stance from the moment of first contact with the patient, along with the following:

1. **Contracting**—A clear agreement regarding the agenda for the current visit, as well as one for the overall nature of the patient–clinician relationship, supports a true partnership. The patient, knowing what to expect, can relax. Trust builds when contracts are completed as negotiated (see Chap. 2).
2. **Listening and tracking**—These are essential to the process of creating a safe environment. "Listening requires being quiet and paying attention to the person who's talking" [1, p. 15]. It requires attending to the patient's words without moving to our heads to plan what we are going to say next [9]. Two classic studies, separated by 15 years, demonstrated the degree to which physicians have difficulty listening. In one study, patients' opening statements were interrupted after an average of 18 s; in the second, the average was 23 s [10, 11]. If patients are not interrupted, their opening statements last only 1–2 min [10].

Tracking refers to the process of commenting on, or asking a question about the patient's immediately preceding statement. It ties the patient's world—including his or her way of understanding the problem—to the clinician's need to obtain the medical data needed for diagnosis [12]. Sometimes the tie is a summarization of what the patient has so far explained. It can also be a short utterance like, "I see," "uh-huh," or an echoing back of a phrase. This gives the patient evidence that the clinician is listening to what he or she just said, and believes it is important.

Patient	The back pain does not let up. I just can't seem to get a handle on it.
Clinician	(*echoing*) You can't get a handle on it.
Patient	The medicine is not helping. It is hard to get all my tasks done when I feel so poorly.

3. **Normalizing**—This increases openness and a sense of emotional safety by acknowledging the universality of a patient's feelings or experience. It often decreases shame [13].

Clinician	Lots of patients forget to take their medication every day. Is that true for you?
Patient	Sometimes I do forget.

4. **Conveying empathy through verbal and nonverbal communication**— Eliciting and responding with empathic statements to the feelings of patients is the topic of Chap. 5. Nonverbal communication of empathy is, perhaps, the more powerful method. Touching a frightened or grieving patient on the elbow or arm can provide powerful comfort and sense of solidarity. (A clinician touching a patient must stay aware of the personal boundary, since touch can feel intrusive to some patients.) It is estimated that 80 % of communication is nonverbal [14].

Nonverbal Tools

Three areas of nonverbal behavior are of particular interest in patient–clinician interactions: proxemics, paralanguage, and kinesics. Both partners in this relationship influence the other via nonverbal communication.

Proxemics is the study of the effect of space and objects in a room and how the patient experiences them. Edward Hall initially described a connection between physical distance and comfort level [15]. Shawn Shea discovered that 90 % of the time interviewers felt most comfortable when seated 4–5 feet apart with the chairs turned 5–10° from a direct line between them. In other words, they did not face each directly in a confrontational manner, but seemed to be facing in the same direction in a collaborative way [16]. Astute clinicians made use of this information to set up the area they will be using for interviewing—a clinic exam room, an office, or even an inpatient room.

Paralanguage refers to how something is said. For instance, consider a busy clinician who rushes. The patient is likely to interpret the nonverbal communication of the clinician as: *I'm a very busy person. I don't have time to listen.* As a result, the patient ignores the clinician's invitation: *Do you have any questions?*

Kinesics refers to movements—body postures, facial expressions, and gestures. The observant interviewer might ask him or herself the following type of question: *Is this patient leaning away and crossing her arms as a signal of withdrawal?* [14] Although nonverbal communication is a rich source of information for the clinician monitoring a patient's sense of emotional safety, it is important not to over interpret an isolated, nonverbal behavior. A patient might lean back to be more comfortable, and not as a signal of withdrawing. Reliability of assessment is increased when nonverbal signals are considered in clusters (for example, a patient leans back, turns head and eyes away, and speaks with a diminished voice—all suggesting withdrawal) [14, 17]. However, trainees do best to focus on one behavior at a time until a level of competent observation is reached [14]. Once a clinician has become skilled recognizing nonverbal communication, he or she has a powerful tool to identify and resolve blocks to effective dialogue, literally as they occur. Carson recommends the use of matching and leading to enhance **rapport** and the patient's feeling of safety [14].

Match—The clinician moves as the patient moves, utilizing one of four nonverbal areas of expression: voice, facial expression, body posture, or gestures. Matching is done subtly in order to avoid bringing attention to the process. The goal is to enter into the patient's world and create synchrony (e.g., a patient drops her head and body posture sags; the clinician leans forward with her head slightly down) [14].

Lead—The clinician gradually moves to a position of safety: relaxed facial and body musculature, arms uncrossed [14]. To the patient, this invitation operates at an unconscious level. In fact, many experienced clinicians match and lead without being aware of the process.

In addition, it is beneficial for clinicians to stay aware of how they phrase their questions. This allows them to use open-ended inquiries when they want their patients to talk freely and focused questions when they want specific details.

Practical Aspects of Formulating Open-Ended Questions and Facilitations

The following categories of verbalization are open-ended—**not easily answered in one or two words** [16].

1. **Facilitations**—Replying *Uh-huh…, I see…* or *Go on…* facilitates the conversation [10]. Head nodding and silence are examples of nonverbal facilitations. They continue the conversation without focusing the interviewee on one topic.

2. **Empathic Summaries**—Stating back to the patient what the clinician has so far heard the patient say in terms of medical data, thoughts, and feelings encourages him or her to say more [2]. The summary is signaled by a stem phrase, such as: *Let me see if a have this right....*

Clinician	Let me see if I have it right. You have chronic pain in your back and shoulder. You feel exhausted much of the time. The problem has worsened during the last 2 months. Your ability to do your daily tasks has been affected. In addition, you are experiencing a lot of stress at home.
Patient	That's right. I am under a lot of stress...

An important component of the summarization is a 5–10 s period of silence at the end to let the empathic summary have an impact on the patient, and give him or her a chance to say more [9]. During this silence, the compassionate clinician can imagine what it is like to be in the patient's position. If a patient does not spontaneously continue telling his or her story, it is useful to follow an empathic summary with a gentle command, one that invites the patient to continue talking.

3. **Gentle Commands**—Gentle commands begin with *Tell me...* or *Describe...*, as in: *Tell me everything about the abdominal pain and diarrhea* or *Describe your relationship with your spouse.* A gentle, curious tone of voice is important, so that the patient feels an invitation to talk. Gentle commands may be the single best tool a clinician possesses to encourage a patient to divulge important matters [16]. Shea points out that adding "can you" to the beginning of a gentle command leads to a terse response as easily as an activation of the patient [16]. It is easy to imagine a rebellious teenager responding: *not much to say* [16, p. 83]. I frequently see a trainee start an inquiry with *Can you tell me...,* instead of simply *Tell me...,* when he or she feels a bit tentative.

4. **Open-Ended Questions**—Open-ended questions begin with "what" or "how" and cannot be answered in one or two words [16]. An example might be: *How will you handle the pressure from your friends*?

However, we note two types of questions that begin with "what" or "how" and are not open-ended: (1) Questions in which the answer set is limited and (2) Questions that begin with "how," ask about the quality of a situation, and can be answered "fine" [16].

What medications are you taking? (The set of medications is limited.)
How is your appetite? (A patient can simply respond: *fine*.)

Incongruence Between Verbal and Nonverbal

One important strategy for creating emotional safety and enhancing a patient's willingness to talk is the confrontation of mixed or incongruent messages. For example, a patient says "fine" to a treatment recommendation but turns his head and eyes away and becomes withdrawn and quiet. Whenever the verbal and nonverbal signals do not match, the nonverbal message more accurately reflects the patient's actual feelings [14]. Confrontation is the process of acknowledging a mixed signal. Confrontation does not mean ignoring the patient's feelings and presenting him or her with the facts [18]. A clinician simply brings the mixed signal into the patient's awareness, allowing the problem to be discussed and potentially resolved. The discrepancy is made overt, while maintaining a positive regard for the patient [14].

Patient	Fine.
Clinician	I know you said fine, but I sensed some hesitation in your voice about taking the medication. Do you have any concerns?

A confrontation can be softened by normalizing the situation: *Lots of people have reservations about starting this type of medication. Is that true for you?*

Key Points

1. Emotional safety is essential to the process of patients feeling free to talk.
2. Contracting, listening, and empathizing all support emotional safety.
3. Nonverbal communication can be used to enhance a patient's sense of safety.
4. Mixed or incongruent messages from patients can be dealt with once they are brought into awareness.

References

1. Platt FW, Gordon GH. Field guide to the difficult patient interview. 2nd ed. Philadelphia, PA: Lippincott Williams and Wilkins; 2004.
2. Lin CT, Platt FW, Hardee JT, Boyle D, Leslie B, Dwinnell B. The medical inquiry: invite, listen, summarize. J Clin Outcomes Manag. 2005;12:415–8.
3. Cox A, Rutter M, Holbrook D. Psychiatric interviewing techniques. V. Experimental study: eliciting factual information. Br J Psychiatry. 1981;139:29–37.
4. Roter DL, Hall JA. Doctors talking with patients/patients talking with doctors: improving communication in medical visits. 2nd ed. Westport, CT: Praeger; 2006.

5. Platt FW, McMath JC. Clinical hypocompetence, the interview. Ann Intern Med. 1979;91:898–902.
6. Linfors EW, Neelon FA. Interrogation and interview: strategies for obtaining clinical data. J R Coll Gen Pract. 1981;31:426–8.
7. Safran DG, Taira DA, Rogers WH, Kosinski M, Ware JE, Tarlov AR. Linking primary care performance to outcomes of care. J Fam Pract. 1998;47:213–20.
8. Headache Study Group of the University of Western Ontario. Predictors of outcome in headache patients presenting to family physicians—a one year prospective study. Headache. 1986;26:285–94.
9. Platt FW, Platt CM. Empathy: a miracle or nothing at all? J Clin Outcomes Manag. 1998;5:30–3.
10. Beckman HB, Frankel RM. The effect of physician behavior on the collection of data. Ann Intern Med. 1984;101:692–6.
11. Marvel MK, Epstein RM, Flowers K, Beckman HB. Soliciting the patient's agenda: have we improved? JAMA. 1999;281:283–7.
12. Mishler EG. The discourse of medicine: dialectics of medical interviews. Norwood, NJ: Ablex; 1984.
13. Shea SC. Improving medication adherence: how to talk with patients about their medications. Philadelphia, PA: Lippincott Williams and Wilkins; 2006.
14. Carson CA. Nonverbal communication. In: Cole SA, Bird J, editors. The medical interview: the three-function approach. 2nd ed. Philadelphia, PA: Mosby; 2000.
15. Hall ET. The hidden dimension. New York, NY: Doubleday; 1966.
16. Shea SC. Psychiatric interviewing: the art of understanding: a practical guide for psychiatrists, psychologists, counselors, social workers, nurses, and other mental health professionals. 2nd ed. Philadelphia, PA: WB Saunders; 1998.
17. Joines V, Stewart I. TA today: a new introduction to transactional analysis. Chapel Hill, NC: Lifespace; 1987.
18. Allmond BW, Tanner JL, Gofman HF. The family is the patient: using family interviews in children's medical care. 2nd ed. Baltimore, MD: Williams and Wilkins; 1999.

Chapter 4
Affirmations

Role Play

Prerequisite role-playing skills for affirmations include **gentle commands, facilitations, listening, tracking, personal story**, and **contracting**.

Role Play: A 47-year-old man with a history of alcohol abuse was recently discharged from the hospital after treatment for pneumonia.

Objectives

1. Obtain a clear contract for the visit.
2. Make one to two descriptive affirmations for any positive choices he is making.

Trainee	Mr. Conn, I know you are here today for follow up of your pneumonia. Is there anything else you want to deal with today?
Patient	I don't think so.
Trainee	One thing I would like to put on the agenda for today is to check on your drinking. Remember, we discussed your use of alcohol when you were in the hospital.
Patient	Yes. That would be okay.
Trainee	Why don't we start with your pneumonia? Tell me how you are doing.
Patient	I'm doing well. I finished up the antibiotic yesterday. I have an occasional cough, but I feel good.

(continued)

Trainee	Do you have any trouble with your breathing?
Patient	No. That seems fine now.
Trainee	How about any general symptoms, such as fever?
Patient	No fever. And my energy is good.
Trainee	Anything else that you have noticed?
Patient	I seem to be a bit nervous. I don't know if it is related, but I haven't had a drink in 11 days.
Trainee	What's that been like for you?
Patient	Not so bad—a little tough at times.
Trainee	How did you decide to stop drinking?
Patient	I think the hospitalization has something to do with it. I want to feel better.
Trainee	Congratulations on your 11 days of sobriety.
Patient	Thanks.
Trainee	Do you have any supports in place, like AA, to help you through this transition?
Patient	I feel like I can do it on my own. I don't like the idea of going to an AA group.
Trainee	You're a pretty independent guy.
Patient	I guess.
Trainee	I'm impressed with your independence and belief in yourself.

Feedback

Faculty	Okay, let's stop. (*to trainee*) What did you like about your interview?
Trainee	I thought I was nonjudgmental. I affirmed the patient for not drinking.
Faculty	Do others have affirmations?
Patient	I experienced you as on my side. I felt comfortable talking to you.
Faculty	I thought you listened well and tracked with the patient. I liked your affirmation of his sobriety.
Trainee	Thanks.
Faculty	Does anybody have options?
Group	(*no response*)
Faculty	I have one option. We know that early sobriety is a high risk time for patients and their families. It is very difficult to get through the turmoil without good psychoeducation and guidance. Instead of

(continued)

affirming his independence, I might ask him for permission to discuss this further, such as, "Would it be okay if we were to discuss using a support system?" If he agrees, I would be curious about his thinking about AA. There are different types of support available. My point is that you can affirm him for making healthy choices—like staying sober—and also confront a possibly unhealthy choice, but in a supportive way.

Trainee That makes sense.
Faculty Are you ready to replay the interview?
Trainee I'm ready.
Faculty Why don't you start from the point you begin to discuss alcohol?

Replay

Trainee How did you decide to stop drinking?
Patient I think the hospitalization has something to do with it. I want to feel better.
Trainee Good for you.
Patient Thanks.
Trainee How were you able to accomplish it?
Patient I just made up my mind.
Trainee Do you plan to use any support groups, like AA, to help you maintain your sobriety?
Patient No. I don't think I need that type of group. I believe I can do it on my own.
Trainee Would it be okay if I tell you a concern I have?
Patient Sure.
Trainee Sobriety is incredibly tough to maintain without the support of others. AA has a long track record of helping folks succeed. What do you know about AA?
Patient I have heard it is like a cult.
Trainee How do you mean "cult"?
Patient I have heard that some people consider AA to be sort of a religious experience. I am not interested in that.
Trainee So, you have learned that some people treat AA like a religion and you are not interested.
Patient Yes.

(continued)

Trainee	I would like to tell you my experience. Would that be okay?
Patient	Okay.
Trainee	I have heard similar comments to yours. I have also heard many more comments from people who have not experienced that. Each group seems to have its own personality. Would you be willing to visit three groups this week before making a judgment?
Patient	I could do that.

Feedback

Faculty	Nice job. I like the way you used my suggestion not to affirm a treatment option with which you did not agree.

Obstacles to Teaching Affirmations

1. Interviewer believes that affirmations are fluff.
2. Interviewer has a lack of experience giving affirmations.

Strategies

1. Use the group process to demonstrate that affirmations are effective in supporting an atmosphere that fosters growth.
2. Educate trainees about the importance of having a 4:1 ratio of positive-to-negative strokes[1] for the maintenance of a healthy environment. Discuss the empirical evidence regarding both the underuse and overuse of affirmations.
3. Give trainees the words to say, such as: *You hold your baby warmly. She looks like she feels very secure in your arms.*

---

[1]Stroke—a term taken from Transactional Analysis, that is defined as a unit of recognition.

Affirmations

Affirmations in this text refer to any verbal or nonverbal behavior that focuses on and shows appreciation for the positive actions or intentions of another person. The positive actions can be small, since any change in a positive direction is generative [1]. The importance of affirmations is modeled in every role-play feedback in this text. Trainees are given affirmations before suggestions for improvement. The faculty mentor builds on the strengths of the trainees.

Affirming patients contributes to a powerful engagement between patient and clinician. Affirmations are the logical consequence of a strength-based model—a philosophical conviction that all people have an okay essence or core. For much of its history, medicine has operated from a deficit model—one that focuses on identifying and eliminating flaws. Take out an inflamed appendix and the patient is cured. It works well when the focus is purely on the physical aspects of a condition. It is an inadequate model for understanding, engaging, and helping patients with the psychosocial aspects of health care. Some examples of this may be coping with a chronic medical condition, becoming motivated to develop a healthier lifestyle, or adhering to a complicated treatment regime. A strength-based, biopsychosocial model is a better model for the modern practice of medicine [2].

Empirical Support for Affirmations

Strong empirical evidence from the study of family and couple relationships, business, and education all support a strength-based approach and the efficacy of affirmations.

The earliest research on the impact of the ways a family interacts and the course of an individual's illness was published in 1963. Patients with schizophrenia had more frequent exacerbations in critical family environments and fewer exacerbations with supportive families [3]. Subsequent studies reported similar results with depression, diabetes, asthma, and a host of other medical conditions [4–6]. Research from John Gottman's experimental lab for couples lends further evidence in support of these findings. He identified a ratio of positive to negative interactions that predicted success in marriages [7]. Couples who communicated with a 5:1 ratio of positive to negative interactions had long-term marriages [7]. Gottman noted that negative interactions regarding their differences were tolerated when positive interactions were frequent.

Synectics, a leading consulting firm for Fortune 500 companies, has had outstanding success helping companies develop creativity and innovation by building on the strengths of those companies [8]. Consultants work with members of the company as they create potential solutions to a problem. Other team members then list the benefits of adopting that potential solution. Only after they list benefits do team members discuss potential flaws with the proposed solution [8]. Listing potential flaws first—a typical approach—has the effect of shutting down innovation.

Education research is replete with examples demonstrating the power of affirmations in shaping behavior [9–11]. A fascinating experiment by a third-grade teacher from Iowa back in 1968 provides a dramatic example of this research. The teacher affirmed blue-eyed children for their intelligence and superiority on the first day of the experiment [12]. These children clearly outperformed the brown-eyed children. When the roles were reversed on the second day of the experiment, brown-eyed children exceeded the blue-eyed children [12]. The evidence is clear. Affirmations have powerful effects on individuals and relationships.

Practical Points

It is useful for clinicians to keep a few practical points in mind when giving affirmations:

1. Follow the patient's lead. If the patient is responding with "yes, but..." it is likely the clinician is too far ahead of the patient. Affirmations would then need to be toned down to match the patient's perspective [1]. This clinician smoothly adjusts her comments to fit the patient's framework:

Clinician	Congratulations on starting a walking program
Patient	Well, I have not been consistent with my exercise.
Clinician	So you have had some success with getting yourself to exercise. It is not the amount you had hoped for. Given all that you are dealing with, how did you decide to start?

2. Some patients will have a filter, developed during their childhood years, which does not allow affirmations to be accepted. One way around this block is to use a *video moment*, rather than a statement that comments on the patient's qualities, such as: *You are a good mother* [11]. This mother may not think of herself as a good mother and reject the compliment. A video moment is a specific description of a behavior that is observed. It is hard to reject because it is not a matter of opinion.

Clinician	I notice you hold your baby warmly. She looks secure and relaxed as she looks into your eyes.
Patient	I like holding her.

3. Giving affirmations does not imply that uncomfortable feelings or problems should be ignored. It is possible to affirm patients for positive motivation and still discuss unhealthy behaviors.

Clinician	Congratulations on maintaining your exercise program.
Patient	Thanks.
Clinician	It is a very positive way to help manage your lung disease. You have got to feel good about that.
Patient	I do.
Clinician	Tell me how you have been doing overall.
Patient	Okay. I feel more energetic since I started walking daily.
Clinician	Joe, one area I would like to check out again today is your drinking, because it can have such a powerful influence on your overall health.
Patient	I'm not doing so hot there.
Clinician	Is it okay if we talk about it for a minute?
Patient	Okay.

4. Affirmations can be very helpful in terms of strengthening a patient's sense of personal responsibility for their health choices and outcomes. Compliments are framed to support patient autonomy—not to please the doctor. The implication is clear and unambiguous: the patient is the one who is in control of his or her actions [1].

Clinician	Getting yourself to begin a walking program, hard as that is, given everything going on in your life right now, has resulted in real improvement in your weight and stamina.
Patient	Thanks.

VS

Clinician	I'm pleased that you started walking and lost weight.
Patient	Thanks.

A clinician new to giving affirmations can be tempted to overdo it. Overdoing affirmations does not magically transform patients [13]. If overdone, patients may perceive the affirmations as disingenuous. Affirmations must be genuine in order to be taken in by the patient and have a positive effect.

Key Points

1. A strength-based approach is an effective framework for dealing with psychosocial issues.
2. Affirmations are a logical consequence of adopting a strength-based clinical approach.
3. Clinicians must reorient themselves in order to take advantage of this powerful engagement tool.

References

1. Walter JL, Peller JE. Becoming solution-focused in brief therapy. Levittown, PA: Brunner/Mazel; 1992.
2. Engel GL. The clinical application of the biopsychosocial model. Am J Psychiatry. 1980;137:535–44.
3. Wynne LC, Singer MT. Thought disorder and family relations of schizophrenics. I. A research strategy. Arch Gen Psychiatry. 1963;9:191–8.
4. Coyne JC. Depression, biology, marriage and marital therapy. Fam Pract. 1987;13:393–407.
5. Campbell TL. The effectiveness of family interventions for physical disorders. J Marital Fam Ther. 2003;29:263–81.
6. McDaniel SH, Campbell TL, Hepworth J, Lorenz A. Family-oriented primary care. 2nd ed. New York, NY: Springer; 2005.
7. Gottman J. Why marriages succeed or fail and how you can make yours last. New York, NY: Fireside; 1995.
8. Mauzy J, Harriman R. Creativity inc: building an inventive organization. Boston, MA: Harvard Business School Press; 2003.
9. Fay J, Funk D. Teaching with love and logic: taking control of the classroom. Golden, CO: Love and Logic Press; 1995.
10. Anderson EM, Maehr ML. Motivation and schooling in the middle grades. Rev Educ Res. 1994;64:287–309.
11. Glasser H, Easley S. Transforming the difficult child: the nurtured heart approach. Nashville, TN: Vaughan Printing; 1998.
12. Peters W. A class divided: then and now. New Haven, CT: Yale University Press; 1987.
13. Widdowson M. Transactional analysis: 100 key points and techniques. New York, NY: Routledge; 2010.

Chapter 5
Eliciting and Responding to Emotions

Role Play

Prerequisite role-playing skills for eliciting and responding to emotions include *gentle commands, facilitations, personal story, attending to nonverbal communication, listening, tracking*, and *contracting*.

Role Play #1:   An 80-year-old woman is telling her story of fading vision. (She responds to empathic statements only if they are accurate.)

Objectives

Make an empathic statement.

Patient	I am having more trouble with my driving. I can't drive at night.
Trainee	Tell me more.
Patient	I think my eyesight is failing. I need large print and strong light to be able to read.
Trainee	I know you have been an avid reader.
Patient	I love to read.
Trainee	You must be very sad about the loss.
Patient	Not really. My mother lost her vision when she got older. I didn't expect my vision to last this long.

The online version of this chapter (doi:10.1007/978-1-4614-7224-7_5) contains supplementary material, which is available to authorized users.

Feedback

Faculty	Let's stop. (*to trainee*) What did you like about your interview?
Trainee	I encouraged her to talk and I gave her space.
Faculty	Yes. And, your pace was excellent. I liked the use of a gentle command, "Tell me more."
Trainee	Thanks.
Faculty	Do you have any options?
Trainee	She did not respond to my empathy.
Faculty	Why do you think she didn't?
Trainee	I don't know.
Faculty	Why don't you ask her?
Trainee	(*to patient*) Why did you not respond to my empathy?
Patient	I wasn't sad. You made an assumption about what I was feeling. **I think it would be important to ask me what I was feeling first**.
Trainee	That makes sense.
Faculty	Lots of people would be sad with loss of vision. She was not. When you ask patients what they are feeling, you can target your empathic statements to their feelings and they are not likely to fall flat. Are you ready to replay the scenario?
Trainee	Yes.

Replay

Patient	I am not able to drive at night nor can I read very well.
Trainee	Tell me more.
Patient	I have read my whole life. Reading is becoming a chore because I need big print.
Trainee	I know reading has always been important to you.
Patient	It has been my passion since I was a child.
Trainee	What has this loss been like for you?
Patient	I expected it at my age. My mother lost her vision at a much younger age.
Trainee	You anticipated the loss and were prepared. How has it affected you emotionally?
Patient	I am a little anxious about how this will affect my day-to-day life.
Trainee	So, you have a little anxiety about how the vision loss will affect your life in a practical way.
Patient	That's right.

Feedback

Faculty	Let's stop. Nice job of eliciting her feelings and then responding with targeted empathy.
Trainee	Thanks.

Role Play #2:　A 62-year-old woman with severe Degenerative Disk Disease has pain and symptoms of spinal stenosis.

Objectives

1. Recognize and acknowledge any changes in the patient's life or losses she has experienced.
2. Elicit her underlying feelings with a direct inquiry.

Trainee	So, tell me how your back is doing.
Patient	I have a lot of pain whenever I stand and walk a little.
Trainee	Tell me about the pain.
Patient	It starts in my buttocks and goes down into my legs, especially on the left side. I'm very limited.
Trainee	Tell me about being limited.
Patient	I used to garden every Saturday and Sunday, but not now. I don't know what to do.
Trainee	What do you feel emotionally as you say that?
Patient	It makes me very angry.
Trainee	*(turns to faculty)* I don't know what to say now.

Feedback

Faculty	What are you feeling as she says she feels very angry?
Trainee	I'm a little anxious. I don't know how to respond. I don't want to make her more upset. I thought she would have just said she was sad about the losses.
Faculty	Good self-awareness on your part. We will come back to this. First, I want to affirm you for noticing her talk about the changes in her life, and then asking her about her feelings. You met the

(continued)

objectives of the role play. I have an idea: our next lesson is on deepening emotions. I could do the demonstration right now and then you could take a shot at responding to this type of answer by helping her deepen her emotional expression. Would you be willing to be the patient for the demonstration? I think it would help you gain a wider perspective.

Trainee   Sure.

Demonstration to Trainees

Faculty   Tell me how your back is doing.
Trainee   I'm still having a lot of pain.
Faculty   Say more.
Trainee   I can only walk for a few minutes before I get pain in my buttocks and down my leg.
Faculty   So, you get pain in your buttocks and leg just by walking a little.
Trainee   Yes. I feel limited in what I can do.
Faculty   What do you feel emotionally?
Trainee   I am very angry about it.
Faculty   Tell me about your anger.
Trainee   I've worked all my life to get to this point. I was hoping I would be able to use this time in my life to do the things I like to do, like gardening. It doesn't seem fair.
Faculty   What are you most upset about?
Trainee   I see people who don't take care of their health not having any problems.
Faculty   No wonder you're feeling angry.
Trainee   I took care of my health all these years.
Faculty   I know. Let me see if I'm hearing you right. You worked hard all your life. You hoped to be able to relax and enjoy your later years, and now you have terrible pain when you try to do activities you like, such as gardening. You feel angry. Is that right? (*silence*)
Trainee   Yes, that's it.
Faculty   Do you have any other feelings besides anger?
Trainee   I'm pretty sad and disappointed. I loved gardening.
Faculty   (*in low voice*) Of course. Tell me about your sadness.
Trainee   It's a big change. I had hoped to learn more about gardening, maybe take a course, and then really get into it. I don't know what I'm going to do.

Feedback

Faculty	Okay. Let's stop the demonstration. (*to trainee*) What did you learn by playing the patient?
Trainee	I see that deepening the affect was helped by your low tone of voice and silence. It definitely helped build rapport. As the patient, I understood better what the loss meant. Talking about anger was not so scary.
Faculty	Are you ready to be the interviewer?
Trainee	Yes

Obstacles to Teaching Eliciting and Responding to Emotions

1. Interviewer believes that a patient is not entitled to feel what he or she is feeling (the circumstances do not justify the feelings).
2. Lack of training in the affective realm (emotional illiteracy) is common.
3. Interviewer attempts to reassure or rescue patients from their feelings.
4. Interviewer fears deepening a patient's emotional experience.
5. Interviewer lacks interest in patient's emotions.
6. Interviewer wants to avoid taking too much time.

Strategies

1. Use reverse role play to allow trainees to experience the difference between having their feelings supported versus having them discounted.
2. Encourage trainees to learn by observing peers, in addition to learning from their own role plays.
3. Teach adverse effects of rescuing.
4. Demonstrate safety and effectiveness of deepening patients' emotions (video or role play).
5. Be patient and respond in nurturing manner to trainees. Evaluate uninterested trainee for possible emotional depletion.
6. Teach closing skills, so the trainee feels confident in his or her ability to structure the interview (see Chap. 7).

Eliciting and Responding to Emotions

Consider two exchanges of dialogue from a primary care practice one afternoon:

A 59-year-old man with tinnitus, present for 4 months.

Patient	What can be done about this constant noise in my ears?
Clinician	There is alternative medicine available online that helps about 50 percent of the time. I'll get you a pamphlet on it.
Patient	Doc, if it doesn't work for me, I don't know what I'll do. I can't stand the fact that the roar is always there in the background.
Clinician	Let's deal with this after you give the medicine a try. There's a fair chance it will help you.

The clinician avoids the patient's feelings, offering reassurance that does not soothe.

A 44-year-old obese woman with diabetes was recently switched from oral hypoglycemic medication to insulin.

Patient	I've not had any real low sugars. The lowest was 70, once.
Clinician	Did it cause you to have any symptoms, such as drowsiness, headache, or sweating?
Patient	No, I didn't feel anything. You know, I remember before I even had diabetes, I didn't have to think about all this stuff. It was really different back then.
Clinician	I imagine it was very different.
Patient	Yes, it sure was.
Clinician	Let me ask you a few more questions about your sugars. How frequently have you been checking your sugars?

The same clinician misses an opportunity to support the second patient altogether because her feelings were not elicited, remaining right under the surface. Both these patients had significant losses. The clinician was not able to help either of the patients with their underlying feelings, despite being a well-motivated clinician.

Clinicians miss as much as 95 % of the available opportunities to respond to their patients' emotions in primary care practice [1–3]. These missed opportunities do matter. When clinicians respond to the emotions of their patients:

1. Health outcomes are improved [4].
2. Patients are more satisfied with their clinician [3].
3. Adherence to treatment recommendations is enhanced [5].

Patients give all kinds of clues to their underlying emotions. We discussed nonverbal clues in Chap. 3, giving special attention to the circumstance of incongruity between the patient's nonverbal and verbal behavior—a circumstance strongly suggestive of underlying feelings. Patients give verbal clues to their underlying feelings when they casually mention life stresses, such as divorce or aging. Repetition of a statement is another common clue, and one that suggests a patient's underlying concerns have not been adequately addressed [2].

Although a clinician could not possibly attend to every clue of every patient, it is important that he or she establishes a safe climate for patients to express their feelings. This is accomplished through a nonjudgmental, accepting approach, clear contracting, verbal and nonverbal empathy, as well as partnering with patients. A number of patients will not express their emotions, especially vulnerable feelings—such as sadness, fear, or hurt—without additional support. Smith and coworkers recommend the use of emotion-seeking skills [6]. These include direct and indirect inquiries.

Direct Inquiry

The following example is both direct and open-ended:

Patient	My back has been killing me. It began hurting right before vacation. The pain prevented me from enjoying any activities with my family. I couldn't sleep well. The only thing that lessens the pain is sitting.
Clinician	How do you feel as you say all that?

Alternatively, the clinician could have asked: *How do you feel, emotionally?* Adding emotionally at the end of the question lets the patient know the clinician is asking about emotions and not somatic feelings. Some patients have not had the experience of others showing an interest in their feelings, and have a strong response.

We know that many patients come to the doctor with specific worries or concerns. A direct, focused inquiry is often all that is needed to make them overt, so that it can be addressed [7].

Patient	My neck and back have been really bothering me. And, I have pain shooting down my arm.
Clinician	What are you most concerned about?
Patient	I'm afraid I have a herniated disc.
Clinician	What about the possibility of a herniated disc concerns you the most?
Patient	I don't want to go through another surgery.

Some patients respond to the use of the word "concern" with an expression of their feelings when they would not do so with the use of the word "worry" [8]. "Concern" is seen as less threatening.

Indirect Inquiry

Indirect ways of eliciting the patient's emotional responses can be useful with guarded patients—people who might experience less threat with indirect inquiries. For example, a patient can be asked what effect the condition has had on the patient and his or her family, since that touches on potential losses [6].

Clinician	How has your diagnosis of spinal stenosis affected your husband?
Patient	Tremendously. He has become so attuned to my needs. (*tears up*)

Often, patients access vulnerable feelings as they report the impact of the illness on their families.

Third-Person Technique

A very useful method of encouraging patients to express feelings, which combines features of both direct and indirect methods, is the third-person technique. The interviewer intuits that a patient is experiencing a certain feeling. He or she then uses the following format: *Lots of patients feel... (the clinician then says the feeling word, such as scared) in this situation. Is that true for you?* Many patients are willing to share their experience once it has been normalized [9].

Clinician's Emotional Literacy

During the course of the patient–clinician relationship, clinicians experience many of the emotions that patients experience: anxiety, sadness, anger, guilt, joy, etc. Some of these emotions are positive; some are negative. Negative feelings (e.g., intense anxiety) have the potential to produce negative interview behaviors, such as over control of the interview, avoidance of psychological issues, superficiality, passivity, or a lack of structuring the interview [6]. These are more likely to result when a clinician is unaware of his or her negative feelings. Trainees commonly lack emotional literacy skills [6]. Whether this is due to the medical culture and training, personality, family background, or other factors, it is a significant deficit. If the clinician does not receive corrective feedback on negative interviewing behaviors, an unhealthy pattern can persist through a career (see Chap. 2) [6].

Emotions have a very important interpersonal function. They guide and motivate behavior by letting each partner know if his or her basic needs for safety, connection, and boundaries are being met. Each feeling contains a message [10]:

Fear—Escape from danger, and get help and reassurance from others.
Anger—Protect ourselves.
Sadness—Withdraw energy, and seek compassion from others.
Joy—Move toward others to share the positive feelings.

Responding to Patients' Feelings

Given the important role emotions play in physician–patient relationships, a thoughtful method for responding to patients' feelings is required. Empathy is fundamental to any effective response, since scientific evidence has demonstrated it to be one of the most important relationship building skills [6]. Patients expressing emotion nonverbally can be invited to express the feelings verbally (e.g., patient who is crying).

Patient	(*tearful*)
Clinician	Put words to your tears.

Cole and Bird recommend the use of two basic types of empathic statements for patients who have expressed their feelings verbally: reflection and normalization. Platt and Gordon suggest a third alternative: the empathic summary.

1. **Reflection** is simply accurately acknowledging the words and emotional experience of another [11].

Patient	I'm anxious about how I will be able to handle these changes.
Clinician	It sounds like you are worried about how all this will affect your life.

OR

Clinician	You look sad.
Patient	I probably am. I hadn't even noticed.

2. **Normalization** lets the patient know his or her feelings are understandable [11].

Patient	Nobody has been able to tell me what my diagnosis is.
Clinician	No wonder you have been frustrated.

3. **Empathic summary**. The empathic summary consists of three parts: a stem, the summary, and a 5–10 s period of silence at the conclusion [12, 13]. The stem is simply a short utterance, such as: *Let me see if I have this right…* or *So…*, that signals to the patient that it is his or her turn to listen. The summary itself can include the medical data, thoughts of the patient about the cause of the illness, values the patient holds, and any feelings expressed by the patient. Summaries vary from a complete reflection of the patient's words to a brief recap of the essential elements. A 5–10 s pause at the conclusion, as we saw in Chap. 3, allows the empathic summary to impact the patient [13]. The pause also gives the clinician time to imagine what it feels like to be in the patient's position. The final part of the empathy cycle is asking and obtaining confirmation from the patient that the clinician has understood accurately [12]. This is very a powerful technique.

Clinician	Let me see if I have it so far. You have chronic back pain. It has gotten much worse in the last month, so much so that you are sleeping poorly and that is really affecting your day-to-day life. You can't concentrate to do your daily tasks. You feel miserable. In addition, you are fearful because nothing you do seems to help. Do I have it right? (*silence for 5–10 seconds*)

Since all three of the above methods repeat what the patient has stated, they are likely to accurately reflect the patient feelings. An annoyed patient is not labeled as angry, which might feel threatening to a patient, who does not want to be angry [11]. However, the level of understanding of the patient's emotional experience may be limited. Obtaining a fuller understanding can be beneficial to both the patient and the clinician.

Deepen Emotional Experience

Patients frequently respond to an inquiry about their feelings with a short statement—one that does not provide any depth. They can be encouraged to expand on their emotional experience. This will lead to a deepening of affect, a greater understanding, and a stronger engagement.

Patient	I feel nervous.
Clinician	Tell me more.
Patient	I've really been anxious since I hurt my back. I haven't been able to provide for my family. I feel lost.
Clinician	You feel lost.
Patient	Yes. I'm the type of person who has always worked. I never took a day off. I'm embarrassed when we can't pay our bills.
Clinician	That has got to be very difficult.

Sometimes patients mention only one feeling, even though they are experiencing more than one feeling. The other emotions may feel more vulnerable to the patient. One way of uncovering those feelings is through direct inquiry: *You have talked about your anxiety, as well as your sense of helplessness. Do you have any other feelings, such as sadness, that go along with this?* Some clinicians are fearful of deepening a patient's emotional experience. They fear that would be intrusive or the patient might become out of control, and the clinician would not know how to contain the feelings. The fact of the matter is that patients control how far they want to go [6]. If a patient does express intense affect, the clinician has tools to help him with those feelings.

Responding to Intense Fear or Sadness

Fear

The purpose of fear is to elicit support and information from the environment. Intense fear arises when a patient views a clinical situation as out of his or her control, such as a new or rapidly worsening clinical condition. Initially, a clinician conveys a sense of support nonverbally with an even tone of voice and relaxed body musculature. This alone helps some patients begin to calm themselves. The next step is to reflect what the patient is communicating verbally or nonverbally [14].

Patient	I don't know how I will handle all this.
Clinician	You sound worried.

It is critical to learn the patient's thoughts, or mental images, that are triggering the intense fear. Patients typically respond to a simple inquiry like: *What concerns you the most about this illness?* [14] Once the patient's thinking has been made overt, he or she is given the needed information. (e.g., *We will use physical therapy, exercises and medications that are effective in easing your type of pain.*) If the fear is realistic, the clinician can express empathy, and continue to support the patient [14].

Patient	So, you are saying I will always have pain when I walk or stand for any length of time.
Clinician	I wish it were different. We will face this condition as a team.

Sadness

Illness involves loss on multiple levels: loss of bodily functions, loss of dignity, loss of independence, loss of purpose, loss of relationships, and loss of dreams. An additional painful loss for patients with a chronic condition is the constant awareness of their condition (e.g., HIV)—of their inability to ever fully enjoy life without worry again [15]. The natural response to loss is sadness, which can be intense in the face of the above losses. Sadness provides important information to the patient. The message to the patient is to mourn the loss, and consolidate a new sense of self. Sadness really hurts. The action of sadness on others invites them to be compassionate: *You look sad* or *Many parents feel a real sense of loss and sadness when they see their child is unable to keep up with others*. Empathy helps soothe the patient's pain.

It is important to respond to someone experiencing deep sadness with a **heart-to-heart exchange**. We grieve and move through loss with our hearts. Some of our responses invite the patient to think, such as: *It is normal to grieve when you experience such a loss*. Thinking responses have value; they provide vital information. However, they do not invite patients to heart-to-heart exchanges. Heart-to-heart responses communicate at an emotional level. A clinician must be willing to be vulnerable in order to respond to a patient at an emotional level. It is important for the clinician to stay present to his or her feelings, and use them as a guide for asking further questions about the patient's experience or making empathic statements. A clinician who makes a self-disclosure—a common response in heart-to-heart exchanges—distracts from the patient [16]. The following examples are responses that keep the focus on the patient's feelings:

- Silence (*as the clinician leans towards the patient*)
- "It is a big loss" (*in a soft voice*)
- "It is heartbreaking" (*in a soft voice*)
- Holding a patient's hand

Closing the Window

Clinicians do need a technique for closing excursions into the emotional arena. Once a patient expresses his or her feelings and has been fully heard (typically 2–7 min), the clinician can utilize an empathic summary to transition the interview back to biomedical data (see Chap. 7 for further development of closing the window) [17].

Key Points

1. The evidence supports improved health outcomes when clinicians support their patients' feelings.
2. Indirect emotion-seeking skills help with guarded patients.
3. Patients are entitled to feel what they feel.
4. Empathic summaries are very effective responses to patients' feelings.

References

1. Suchman AL, Markakis K, Beckman HB, Frankel R. A model of empathic communication in the medical interview. JAMA. 1997;277:678–82.
2. Levinson W, Gorawara-Bhat R, Lamb J. A study of patient clues and physician responses in primary care and surgical settings. JAMA. 2000;284:1021–7.
3. Putnam SM, Lipkin M. The patient-centered interview: research support. In: Lipkin M, Putnam SM, Lazare A, editors. The medical interview: clinical care, education, and research. New York, NY: Springer; 1995.
4. Stewart MA. Effective physician-patient communication and health outcomes: a review. CMAJ. 1995;152:1423–33.
5. Rollnick S, Miller WR, Butler CC. Motivational interviewing in health care: helping patients change behavior. New York, NY: The Guilford; 2008.
6. Fortin A, Dwamena FC, Frankel RM, Smith RC. Smith's patient-centered interviewing: an evidence-based method. 3rd ed. New York, NY: McGraw Hill; 2012.
7. Korsch BM, Aley EF. Pediatric interviewing techniques: current pediatric therapy. Sci Am. 1973;3:1–42.
8. Bass LW, Cohen RL. Ostensible versus actual reasons for seeking pediatric attention: another look at the parental ticket of admission. Pediatrics. 1982;70:870–4.
9. Gould RK, Rothenberg MB. The chronically ill child facing death: how can the pediatrician help. Clin Pediatr. 1973;12:447–9.
10. Widdowson M. Transactional analysis: 100 key points and techniques. New York, NY: Routledge; 2010.
11. Cole SA, Bird J. The medical interview: the three function approach. 2nd ed. Philadelphia, PA: Mosby; 2000.
12. Lin CT, Platt FW, Hardee JT, Boyle D, Leslie B, Dwinnell B. The medical inquiry: invite, listen, summarize. J Clin Outcomes Manag. 2005;12:415–8.
13. Platt FW, Platt CM. Empathy: a miracle or nothing at all? J Clin Outcomes Manag. 1998;5:30–3.
14. Egener B. Responding to strong emotions. In: Novack DH, Clark WD, Daetwyler C, Saizow DB, editors. doc.com – an interactive learning resource for healthcare communication [Internet]: American Academy on Communication in Healthcare/Drexel University College of Medicine; Accessed on 03/12/12; http://www.AACHonline.org
15. Shea SC. Improving medication adherence; how to talk with patients about their medications. Philadelphia, PA: Lippincott Williams and Wilkins; 2006.
16. McDaniel SH, Beckman H, Morse D, Seaburn D, Silberman J, Epstein R. Physician self–disclosure in the primary care visits: enough about you, what about me? Arch Intern Med. 2007;167:1321–6.
17. Branch WT, Malik TK. Using 'windows of opportunities' in brief interviews to understand patients' concerns. JAMA. 1993;269:1667–8.

Chapter 6
Uncovering Self-Diagnosis

Role Play

Prerequisite role-playing skills for the explanatory mode include **gentle commands, listening, tracking**, *clarifying*, **contracting**, *eliciting* and *responding to emotions*, and **personal story**.

Role Play: A 28-year-old woman has had Crohn's disease since adolescence. She is currently a graduate student. Her medical condition has deteriorated over the last 18 months, although she is currently stable. This is her initial visit to a new clinician.

Objective

Obtain the patient's theory of illness.

Trainee	Before we get started with your medical concerns, would you take a minute to tell me about yourself personally, so I can get to know you.
Patient	I am 28 years old and single. I am a graduate student in psychology. That has been my dream since I was 8 years old. My mother was a psychiatrist in private practice. I finish my training in 6 months.

(continued)

J. Binder, *Primary Care Interviewing: Learning Through Role Play*,
DOI 10.1007/978-1-4614-7224-7_6, © Springer Science+Business Media New York 2013

Trainee	Congratulations. So you are finishing graduate school in 6 months. Tell me more about yourself.
Patient	Well, I have worked hard to get to this point. As you know, I have Crohn's disease. I have had a rough couple of years. I should have graduated already.
Trainee	I imagine that has been a real disappointment.
Patient	It has been. On the other hand, I feel the professors and school have been understanding and supportive.
Trainee	So, you have felt supported by the school accepting the demands of your illness. This might be a good time to hear about your illness. You say you have had a rough couple of years. Tell me more.
Patient	I have been hospitalized two times in the last year and a half. I've had a lot of abdominal pain and trouble maintaining my weight.
Trainee	What is your sense about the reason for your increased difficulty?
Patient	I don't know.
Trainee	*(turns to faculty)* I don't know where to go from here.
Faculty	I think you are on the right track. I would persist with another inquiry, maybe "I know you don't know for sure, but if you had to guess, what might you say?"
Trainee	*(turns to patient)* Okay, so, if you had to make a guess, even though you don't know for sure, what might you say?
Patient	To tell you the truth, I think it could be all the stress of graduate school, and how I have handled the stress.
Trainee	What do you mean?
Patient	I've gotten very anxious, even panicky at times. I'm sure that is not good for the Crohn's.
Trainee	So, you see the exacerbations of your Crohn's disease as a direct result of how you have managed your anxiety.
Patient	That's mostly it.

Feedback

Faculty	Let's stop. *(to patient)* Will you tell the interviewer what you experienced positively during the interview?
Patient	I experienced a lot of positives. I thought you *(trainee)* really wanted to hear my perspective. You took time to get to know me and what I thought.
Faculty	Other affirmations?

(continued)

Trainee #2	I like the way you took time to ask for help when you were stuck.
Faculty	In addition to the above, I noticed that you expressed empathy for her with, "I imagine that has been a real disappointment." I liked the use of the word *imagine*. You also asked her for her explanation of the worsening of her illness.
Trainee	Thanks.
Faculty	Does anybody have options?
Group	(*no response*)
Faculty	I have already given you my one option, which is to be persistent in obtaining the patient's theory of illness. Understanding the patient's theory of illness is important for several reasons. It helps the clinician understand his or her patient's experience of illness better. And, it allows the clinician to partner with the patient on a treatment plan. For example, let's say the clinician discovers the above patient believes that maintaining herself on medication for Crohn's disease is a sign that she is not managing her anxiety well. As a test, she has stopped her immunosuppressant medication for Crohn's. That would be vital information.

Obstacles to Teaching Uncovering Self-Diagnosis

1. Interviewer does not recognize the importance of the patient's theory of illness.
2. Interviewer gives up when a patient does not provide his or her theory of illness immediately.

Strategies

1. Educate trainees regarding the patient's perspective and how it impacts engagement and treatment.
2. Coach trainees to persist during role play.

Uncovering Self-Diagnosis and Other Health Beliefs

A friend of mine told me the following story on his return from a mission trip to an underdeveloped country.

A middle-aged woman arrived at the clinic, claiming to be a werewolf. Through an interpreter, she explained that, in the evening she stumbled when she attempted to walk, appearing wild to her family and neighbors. She was incorrectly labeled a werewolf, but the patient adopted the community's belief about her condition. On physical exam, this woman had a significant peripheral neuropathy. She compensated with visual clues, which were not available to her after the evening sunset. The clinician and patient talked about all this and created a practical plan together to help her in the evenings.

This patient and physician had different ways of interpreting the same symptom. It is a dramatic example. It is not an anomaly. Many patients hold beliefs about their illnesses that cause them unnecessary emotional suffering [1]. Erroneous patient beliefs about illness present common barriers to effective treatment.

Understanding the meaning of an illness to a patient has several distinct advantages for clinicians:

1. Engagement is strengthened by deepening the clinician's understanding of his or her patient.
2. The clinician can more readily partner with his or her patient and avoid futile treatment plans.

Explanatory Model

It is probably safe to assume that all patients have imagined thoughts about their symptoms and the meaning of those symptoms. If we do not learn about those beliefs, we may end up puzzled by our patients' behavior and label it as resistant [2]. A classic pattern in pediatrics is observing parents who are more concerned than the history and physical findings seem to warrant [3].

Mother	My baby's been real congested for 2 days.
Clinician	Tell me about the trouble breathing.
Mother	The congestion is making it hard for her to breathe.
Clinician	Is it affecting how much of the bottle she drinks?
Mother	No, she's drinking 6 ounces at a time, but she gags and chokes.
Clinician	Tell me about the choking.
Mother	Sometimes the mucous gets stuck in her throat.
Clinician	What concerns you the most?
Mother	That she is choking and can't catch her breath.
Clinician	So you are concerned that she won't be able to catch her breath. What a scary thought. We will talk about that as soon as I finish examining her.

Many adult patients also imagine the cause or course of their illnesses to be worse than the reality [1]. Fears can only be addressed when they have been brought out into the open. Kleinman et al. suggest the following nonjudgmental questions [4]:

What do you think is causing your problem?
Why do you think it started when it did?
What do you think your sickness does to you? How does it work?
How has it affected you physically? Personally?
How severe is your sickness? How long do you think it will last?
What are the chief problems your sickness has caused for you?
What concerns you most about your sickness?

Inquiring into the patient's theory of illness can be integrated into the interview any time after rapport has been established. It does not have to take much time. It occasionally requires gentle persistence [2]. In the following example, persistence helps the clinician uncover that the patient is not adhering to his treatment for hypertension, which then can be approached as a problem to be solved together. Poor adherence to treatment occurs one-third of the time in patients with chronic conditions [5].

Clinician	I'd like to discuss your blood pressure control. Tell me how it looks to you.
Patient	Not so good from the reading today.
Clinician	Let's take a second to make sure we are on the same page. Tell me your thoughts about the cause of your hypertension.
Patient	I don't really know. I guess it runs in my family.
Clinician	That's true. Do you have a general view about how that works in your body?
Patient	Not really.
Clinician	Some people have an idea that tension, from the word hypertension, must play an important role. Is that part of your thinking?
Patient	Actually, it is. I figure when I'm tense, my blood pressure must be high.
Clinician	Tell me more.
Patient	When I'm having increased stress in my life, I'm more likely to make sure I take my medication.
Clinician	How about times when you feel calmer?
Patient	I'm not as compulsive about taking my medication. I guess I'm thinking it is not as important at those times.
Clinician	Let me see, if I understand you correctly... You believe genetics and stress play important roles in your hypertension. You are careful to take your medication when your overall stress level is high, not so careful at other times. Do I have it right?
Patient	Yes, that's it.
Clinician	Would you be interested in hearing what we have learned about the control of hypertension from recent studies?
Patient	Sure.

It took only a bit of persistence to get at this patient's beliefs. Some patients will need greater persistence, and even an acknowledgement of our ignorance [2].

Clinician	I still don't have a full picture. Would you help me understand better how this looks to you?
Patient	I think...

A patient's explanatory model of illness strongly influences the patient's overall perspective of his or her illness. It is also informed by the patient's culture, socioeconomic status, spiritual beliefs, personal stresses, and issues [6]. Patients respond in diverse ways to an illness: as a challenge to be fought, as a punishment from God to be endured, as a loss to be grieved, or even as an opportunity from which to grow [7]. Patients assign a symbolic meaning to their illness. In the following exchange, the internist explores the symbolic meaning of a recent myocardial infarction to a patient.

Clinician	What are your thoughts about your recent hospitalization?
Patient	How do you mean?
Clinician	Lots of people who have had a heart attack begin to ask themselves questions, such as, "How did it happen?" or "Why did it happen?"
Patient	I have done that. I sometimes think I brought it on myself. I kept thinking I would start to take better care of myself by eating healthy and taking my blood pressure medications like I was supposed to take them... I never did.
Clinician	What do you feel emotionally as you say all that?
Patient	I feel terrible, guilty.
Clinician	Sounds like you are being hard on yourself.
Patient	Doc, I believe I deserve it.

If our job as physicians is to help patients feel and function better, then it is essential for us to understand the meaning of the illness to the patient, symbolically and functionally.

Key Points

1. Patients often hold beliefs about their illness that are mistaken and lead to unnecessary suffering.

2. It is important to identify those beliefs, so that misunderstandings can be addressed and potentially resolved.
3. Understanding the meaning of a patient's illness strengthens engagement.
4. Taking the patient's theory of illness into account allows the clinician to effectively partner with the patient on a treatment plan.
5. Clinicians become puzzled by patient and family behaviors when they do not understand the meaning of the illness to the patient and family [2].
6. The patient's perspective includes both the explanatory model and the symbolic and functional meaning of the illness.

References

1. Martin AR. Exploring patient beliefs: steps to enhancing physician-patient interaction. Arch Intern Med. 1983;143:1773–5.
2. Platt FW, Gordon GH. Field guide to the difficult patient interview. 2nd ed. Philadelphia, PA: Lippincott Williams and Wilkins; 2004.
3. Bass LW, Cohen RL. Ostensible versus actual reasons for seeking pediatric attention: another look at the parental ticket of admission. Pediatrics. 1982;70:870–4.
4. Kleinman A, Eisenberg L, Good B. Culture, illness, and care. Clinical lessons from anthropologic and cross-cultural research. Ann Intern Med. 1978;88:251–8.
5. Sackett DL, Snow JC. The magnitude of compliance and noncompliance. In: Haynes R, Sackett DL, Taylor D, editors. Adherence in health care. Baltimore, MD: John Hopkins University Press; 1979.
6. Betancourt JR. Cross-cultural medical education: conceptual approaches and frameworks for evaluation. Acad Med. 2003;78:560–9.
7. Caress AL, Luker KA, Owens RG. A descriptive study of meaning of illness in chronic renal disease. J Adv Nurs. 2001;33:716–27.

Chapter 7
Structure

Role Play

Prerequisite interviewing skills for role-playing structure include **gentle commands**, **listening, tracking**, *clarifying*, **contracting, empathic summary**, and **referred gate**.

Role Play: A 57-year-old mother of two adult children presents with back and knee pain, along with chronic fatigue. Her own mother is in the middle stage of Alzheimer's Dementia, requiring an increased level of care.

Objectives

1. Listen and empathize with the patient's feelings of depletion and sadness.
2. Use a transitional statement (e.g., empathic summary or referred gate) to guide the interview back to the patient's symptoms.

Trainee	Mrs. Lowe, what would you like to put on the agenda for today?
Patient	My back is acting up.
Trainee	Anything else?
Patient	My left knee is hurting.
Trainee	Anything else?
Patient	No, but I do have a question about my mom.
Trainee	Do you want to start with that?
Patient	My mom won't let us bathe her any more. She fights us when we try to clean her.

(continued)

Trainee	That sounds difficult. Tell me more.
Patient	She seems to be fearful of the water, especially when we try to wash her hair.
Trainee	How have you dealt with it?
Patient	Not well. I try to reassure her. That doesn't work. Sometimes I get frustrated.
Trainee	What is the toughest part for you?
Patient	I hate to see her like this.
Trainee	Of course.
Patient	(*crying softly*)
Trainee	It's such a big loss for you.
Patient	Yes.
Trainee	(*silence*)
Patient	What do you think I should do?
Trainee	That's a great question. Let me think about this some more. As a start, you might call the Alzheimer's Association. It's a common problem of families who have a member with Alzheimer's and they are usually very helpful.
Patient	Okay.
Trainee	Mrs. Lowe, earlier you said your back was hurting. Tell me about that.

Feedback

Faculty	Let's stop. Does anyone have affirmations?
Patient	I thought you listened well to me and supported me. I felt ready to discuss my back problem when you shifted the interview to my symptoms.
Trainee #2	I liked the way you referred back to her earlier statement. It was clear that you were listening to her.
Faculty	I thought you did a nice job of staying with her feelings. You didn't rush. Then, you used a referred gate to move the interview along smoothly.
Trainee	Thanks.
Faculty	Does anybody have options?
Group	(*no response*)
Faculty	Okay. Good job.

Obstacles to Teaching Structuring

1. Interviewer believes that being a good listener means not intervening at all.
2. Trainee believes that guiding or structuring statements will offend patients.
3. Trainee believes a closed-ended, controlling style is needed to manage time.

Strategies

1. Use reverse role play so that the trainee experiences the ability of the clinician to listen and empathize, as well as guide the interviewee.
2. Utilize self-awareness and group discussion to help trainees see the connection between their family of origin and being nonassertive.
3. Empathize with the controlling trainee's efforts to structure and get the data. Help him or her learn to integrate the tools from Chaps. 1–7 through repeated role plays.
4. Teach trainees how controlling styles miss important data.

Structuring

Chaotic and meandering interviews are inefficient and do not accomplish the overall tasks of the session. Without a clear structure, one or more parts of the interview will be compromised, as well as the goals of that phase of the interview. A second, equally important reason to organize a medical interview is patient perception. One of the ways patients evaluate physician expertise is by assessing their leadership and thoroughness demonstrated when questioning patients about symptom details [1]. Wandering interviews lead to decreased patient trust, as well as incomplete details regarding symptoms. Trust is one of the key overall goals of the medical interview, since health outcomes relate to trust, among other variables [2].

A structured interview certainly should not be equated with a high-control, closed-ended style of interviewing—a style that has been demonstrated to miss important data [3–5]. Structuring a medical interview simply refers to the existence of clear boundaries between parts of the interview. Within that structure, patients can be encouraged to open up, tell their stories, express their feelings, and provide a theory of causation. Physicians are then able to fill in missing medical details, weaving in open-ended focused questioning. In other words, the interview has flexibility. The more experience a clinician gains, the more he or she will be able to move smoothly between the parts of the interview. Trainees cannot gain this experiential knowledge quickly. They must learn the content of medical illnesses and how to use the interviewing tools discussed in this text. Integration of these skills takes time, practice, and constructive feedback.

The tasks of the three phases of the medical interview are outlined below, followed by a discussion of interviewing strategies and techniques that smoothly guide the interviewer through the three phases.

Tasks of Interview

Opening Phase

1. Create a working relationship with the patient, one based on mutual respect and trust.
2. Establish emotional safety.
3. Check your own internal emotional experience.
4. Activate the patient to give his or her perception of the problem.
5. Evaluate the process of the interview [1].
6. Obtain the patient's full agenda, organize and prioritize it, and then explain your plan for the rest of the interview to the patient [6, p.12].

Middle Phase

1. Obtain a full and accurate data base [7].
2. Maintain engagement.

Concluding Phase

1. Check that patient understands the condition or problem.
2. Provide information about the condition in chunks.
3. Attend to the patient's emotional reaction.
4. Correct any of the patient misperceptions about the condition.
5. Have patient restate what they have heard the clinician say so that patient and clinician have a shared understanding.
6. Partner with the patient to develop forward steps.

Structuring Strategies

It is up to the clinician to create and maintain an organized, yet engaged interview. He or she may use a few basic strategies: preparation, time management, contracting, making the process overt, and guiding movement through the interview with transitional statements.

Preparation

A plan can avoid many of the common interruptions to the medical interview. These interruptions, such as routine telephone calls or cell phones ringing, fracture the flow and organization of the interview. Discussions with staff and signs posted in the office can easily prevent these disruptions. Even completing computer forms on each patient can be managed without interrupting the flow of the key parts of patients' histories.

Use of Computers

It is important for clinicians who use computers in the exam room to first obtain an agreement with the patient or family to use the computer [8].

Clinician	From time to time, I will be entering information into the computer. Is that okay with you?
Patient	Sure.
Clinician	If it starts to bother you, will you let me know?
Patient	I will.

Since it is impossible to simultaneously type on the computer and be fully engaged with the patient, information must be entered into the computer intermittently. One way of accomplishing this is to perform key parts of the history in the usual fashion (e.g., attend solely to the patient, jotting down an occasional note, during the personal story, contracting process, history of present illness, etc.) and then stop to enter the data into the computer. The clinician maintains engagement while entering data into the computer by maintaining intermittent eye contact and attending to nonverbal behavior [9]. This means the patient has to be seated in a location accessible to the clinician and computer.

Time Management

A clear structure begins with good time management. Time management is the clinician's responsibility—not the patient's. The seasoned clinician stays aware of the time available for the visit and the amount he or she wants to allot to each phase of the interview. The opening phase can vary extensively, but an average time to complete it is 3–5 min. Time spent in the middle phase parallels the complexity and number of problems contracted in the opening phase. It is important to leave enough time to complete an unhurried concluding phase, perhaps 5 min on average.

Starting and ending appointments late are often accepted as the price patients must pay for being able to see the doctor. This discounts patients and clinicians. The metacommunication received by patients when appointments routinely run late is: *Your needs and plans are not important.* Chronically rushing adds tension to the lives of physicians, and it negatively impacts their ability to be fully present to each patient.

Contract

This is a reminder to secure a specific contract. Completing that contract creates a clear structure for each medical visit. Patient security is increased by knowing what to expect. (See Chap. 2 for further development of the contracting process.)

Make the Process Overt

Clinicians possess a powerful, exquisitely simple method for helping a patient stay on track and accomplish the goals of the interview. Tell the patient what is needed and why it is needed.

Clinician	Mrs. Williams, it sounds like you have seen a number of physicians about your headaches over the years. I would like to hear about that a little bit later. It will help me get a better understanding of your illness if you would first tell me more about the symptoms—headache, nausea, that sort of thing. Would you please start at the beginning and tell me all about your symptoms.
Patient	Sure.

A corollary of **making the process overt** is for the clinician to ask permission— to ask further questions on a sensitive topic, offer a treatment recommendation, or change the subject. In effect, he or she guides the interview by **introducing** this question.

Guiding[1]

Guiding the medical interview takes on primary importance in the second phase, since the clinician must gather a large amount of data from different regions. A simple, yet elegant, technique for guiding patients is echoing back only part of their most recent utterance. This emphasis invites them to focus on that phrase [10].

Patient	I have been having headaches almost every day. It is like someone is squeezing my head. The Ibuprofen relieves the headache temporarily. Sometimes they bother me so much I feel nauseous.
Clinician	(*echoing*) Nauseous.
Patient	Yes, but only when the headaches are severe.

The most efficient method of gathering data is to fully assess one region (e.g., symptom descriptors for nausea) before moving to the next region [1]. In addition, it is easier to remember what details are needed for diagnosis when they are grouped together. If a patient mentions an item outside the region, the clinician can jot down a note to remind him or herself to return to the topic later. When the clinician is finished with a region, he or she has a number of options for transitioning to the next region. These transitional statements solidify the conversational feel of the history and help the patient stay activated.

The following **transition** statements allow the clinician to guide the interview to specific regions.

Empathic Summary—This is a recap of the data and experience narrated by the patient. It eases transition to the next topic [11].

Clinician	Let me see if I heard you correctly… You have had headaches for years. They have become worse in the past month. They usually get worse as the day goes on. Ibuprofen helps for a while. You don't think you are experiencing any more stress than usual. You are concerned about the possibility of a brain tumor because they are occurring daily.
Patient	That's right.
Clinician	Now, tell me any symptoms that you have noticed with the headaches.

---

[1] Shawn Shea defines a region as a part of the interview that stays on a topic for several sentences in a row or more. A gate is a transition statement that joins two different regions of the history.

Empathic summaries have long been used by experienced clinicians in private practice to transition back to the presenting symptoms after taking anywhere from 2 to 7 min to discuss a personal, emotional, or family issue that arises during the visit [12]. It allows them to be empathic and stay on time. Branch and Malik labeled this as "closing the window."

Referred Gate—A clinician refers back to one earlier statement made by the patient and uses that to move to a new topic [1]. This powerful technique allows the clinician to enter a new or old region **at will**—even an awkward one, such as the mental status exam—as in the following exchange [1]:

Patient	I took Ibuprofen for the headache, but it didn't help much.
Clinician	Uh-huh. Earlier you said that your headache today was severe and that you were having trouble concentrating. I would like to ask you a few questions to check your concentration and memory. Some of the questions will be basic, and others more difficult.

Third-Person Technique—This technique—an interesting corollary of the referred gate—references the general category of people presenting with this symptom. Instead of referring back to a specific statement made by a particular patient, the third-person technique is used to ask questions about features of the symptom that other patients have experienced [13].

Patient	I haven't noticed any new stresses.
Clinician	Lots of times people can be unaware of the stresses they are handling. We have learned that some people who are experiencing the type of headaches you have can also be dealing with worries or even a depression. Would it be okay if I ask you about those topics? (*third-person technique*)
Patient	Sure.
Clinician	Do people say you are the type of person that tends to worry?
Patient	My husband would say I am a worrier.

Implied Gate—The interviewer simply moves the interviewee to a new topic that appears to be generally related to the first topic [1]. In the following vignette, the interviewer guides the interviewee from panic to assessment of depression.

Patient	The anxiety attacks come out of nowhere.
Clinician	I imagine that is frightening. Let me see if I have this right. You have noticed sudden episodes of feeling panicky one or two times a week over the last 3–4 weeks. The episodes come out of nowhere and last about 45 minutes.
Patient	Yes.
Clinician	Have you ever before experienced episodes like this?
Patient	No, never.
Clinician	What about your mood—have you felt depressed, blue or had difficulty enjoying activities that you usually enjoy?
Patient	Maybe.
Clinician	Tell me what you have noticed.

One type of patient, commonly seen in primary care, the wandering patient, requires a specific structuring approach.

Structuring a Wandering Patient

Progressive structuring is the technique of choice for wandering patients [1]. The first task involves listening to the patient, perhaps for 3–5 min. Any signs of clinician frustration should be avoided, since it will be sensed by the patient, increasing anxiety and wandering. **The clinician must take the time to understand the symbolic meaning of what the patient is saying, and acknowledge his or her feelings before structuring**. Otherwise, the patient is likely to feel discounted [1]. The clinician begins structuring by simply telling the patient what is needed. The following exchange of dialogue is **4 min** into a visit with Mrs. Williams, the patient with recurrent headaches. The clinician has listened quietly and responded compassionately to her feelings during this opening phase.

Clinician	I would like to now ask you some doctor-type questions about the headaches.
Patient	Okay.
Clinician	Tell me about the frequency of the headaches.
Patient	My headaches are unpredictable. My sister was visiting from North Carolina last week and I got a horrible headache the day she was leaving. She is not able to visit very often. She has two

(continued)

> children who are hyperactive. As I was telling you previously, I worry about her. She and I have always been very close. In fact, when we were children, we were inseparable. We still talk on the phone almost every day.
>
> **Clinician** Mrs. Williams, the circumstances in which headaches occur are important. We will return to it later. For now, it would help me to understand the characteristics of the headaches themselves. Tell me how frequent the headaches have been over the last four weeks.

If further structuring becomes necessary, it can be accomplished by establishing a **new contract**. The patient and clinician make an agreement to keep the interview on track [1].

> **Clinician** I believe it is important for us to focus on one topic at a time, so that I can get a clear understanding of your headaches. I hear your concern about your sister and I promise we will deal with it later. If we wander away from the headaches, I will bring us back. Is that okay?

Rarely, the clinician is faced with a runaway process. Fred Platt suggests touching the speaker in a nonvulnerable spot, such as the elbow and saying the patient's name out loud to gain control of the process. Once the patient slows down, the clinician continues to weave open and closed questions into the dialogue [14]. "Clinicians often believe that they must resort to closed-ended questions in order to control a runaway interview. That is a medical myth. Yes, we need to control the process, but we still want to allow the patient or parent the freedom to tell his or her story."(Platt, March 2010)

Family

Establishing a structure for family visits parallels the process discussed for individuals. It is even more important to have clear boundaries because of the potential for greater chaos and disruption with multiple people present in the room. Although families present more challenges, they also allow for a whole new set of interventions to guide the interview. Methods of structuring family visits are discussed in Chap. 13.

Key Points

1. Trainees need time and supervision to learn the complex skill of guiding the medical interview, while simultaneously maintaining a patient focus.
2. Clinicians are more likely to invite patients to talk openly and respond to expressions of emotion once they develop the skills that allow them to control the flow of the interview.
3. Structuring family interviews is crucial and calls for a different set of skills than those needed for individual patients (see Chap. 13).
4. Family-of-origin issues have a powerful effect on how trainees structure interviews. Some can be controlling, and others reluctant to guide at all. These issues can be addressed in small group discussions (see Introduction).

References

1. Shea SC. Psychiatric interviewing: the art of understanding: a practical guide for psychiatrists, psychologists, counselors, social workers, nurses, and other mental health professionals. 2nd ed. Philadelphia, PA: WB Saunders; 1998.
2. Safran DG, Taira DA, Rogers WH, Kosinski M, Ware JE, Tarlov AR. Linking primary care performance to outcomes of care. J Fam Pract. 1998;47:213–20.
3. Platt FW, McMath JC. Clinical hypocompetence: the interview. Ann Intern Med. 1978;9:898–902.
4. Cox A, Rutter M, Holbrook D. Psychiatric interviewing techniques. V. Experimental study: eliciting factual information. Br J Psychiatry. 1981;139:29–37.
5. Linfors EW, Neelon FA. Interrogation and interview strategies for obtaining clinical data. J R Coll Gen Pract. 1981;31:426–8.
6. Binder J. Pediatric interviewing: a practical, relationship-based approach. New York, NY: Humana Press; 2010.
7. Cole SA, Bird J. The medical interview: the three function approach. 2nd ed. Philadelphia, PA: Mosby; 2000.
8. Ventres WB, Frankel RM. Patient-centered-care and electronic health records: it's still about the relationship. Fam Med. 2010;42:364–6.
9. Frankel R. Effects of exam-room computing on clinician-patient communication: a longitudinal qualitative study. J Gen Intern Med. 2005;20:677–82.
10. Fortin A, Dwamena FC, Frankel RM, Smith RC. Smith's patient-centered interviewing: an evidence-based method. 3rd ed. New York, NY: McGraw Hill; 2012.
11. Coulehan JL, Platt FW, Egener B, Frankel R, Lin CT, Lown B, et al. "Let me see if I have this right...": words that help build empathy. Ann Intern Med. 2001;135:221–7.
12. Branch WT, Malik TK. Using 'windows of opportunities' in brief interviews to understand patients' concerns. JAMA. 1993;269:1667–8.
13. Gould RK, Rothenberg MB. The chronically ill child facing death: how can the pediatrician help. Clin Pediatr. 1973;12:447–9.
14. Platt FW, Gordon GH. Field guide to the difficult patient interview. 2nd ed. Philadelphia, PA: Lippincott Williams and Wilkins; 2004.

Chapter 8
Accuracy

Role Play

Prerequisite interviewing skills for role-playing accuracy include **gentle commands**, **listening**, *tracking*, **personal story**, **contracting**, *clarifying, eliciting, and responding to emotions*, and *obtaining* **theory of illness**.

Role Play #1:   A 83-year-old man visits his primary care clinician for a routine follow up. He has congestive heart failure and insomnia.

Objectives

1. Agree to a clear contract for the visit.
2. Clarify any vague terms or statements.

Trainee	Mr. Rollins, what is most important for you to accomplish in today's visit?
Patient	I'm here for a checkup and to get blood work.
Trainee	Is there anything you want to make sure we talk about during our time together?
Patient	I'm a little more tired.
Trainee	Tell me what you mean by "a little more tired."
Patient	I feel buggy—out of sorts during the day.
Trainee	By "buggy," do you mean you feel irritable?
Patient	Yes.
Trainee	Are you feeling sleepy during the day?

(continued)

Patient	I don't sleep well.
Trainee	It sounds like the problem is being sleepy during the day?
Patient	Yes.
Trainee	Anything else you want to talk about?
Patient	My wife thinks I'm slowing down. She is concerned that I don't move around enough.
Trainee	What do you think?
Patient	I do watch a lot of television.
Trainee	What is the reason for that?
Patient	It is just so hard to move about.
Trainee	Uh-huh, tell me about it.
Patient	I just sit in front of the television. Trying to doing anything feels like a big chore.
Trainee	That must be difficult for you. Do you get short of breath when you walk around, or do you mean your motivation is low, or something else?
Patient	I get winded when I walk.
Trainee	Mr. Rollins, it sounds like there are two things for us to discuss. One is trouble sleeping. The other is getting short of breath with activity. Is there anything else?
Patient	No.
Trainee	Why don't we start with the shortness of breath? Tell me about it.
Patient	I can't walk very far or fast.
Trainee	How far would you say you walk: 10, 50, or 100 feet before your breathing gets affected?
Patient	Maybe 100 feet.
Trainee	What happens then?

Feedback

Faculty	Okay, let's stop here. Does anyone have affirmations?
Trainee #2	I thought you clarified the vague words the patient used like "buggy."
Trainee #3	I like how careful you were to make sure you understood him.
Faculty	Will you tell her what you noticed?
Trainee	You (*trainee*) persisted. You kept asking him questions until you understood what that his chief complaints were: insomnia and dyspnea on exertion.

(continued)

Faculty	I agree. I also like the way you set up a clear, crisp contact for the session.
Trainee	Thanks.
Faculty	Does anybody have options?
Group	No.
Faculty	One possibility that occurred to me was the opportunity to include his wife at future visits. He mentioned her concern about his activity level. She could be a rich source of accurate information, as well as a support. You could talk with him about the importance of including family with his type of medical problems, and ask him if he would be willing to invite his wife to accompany him for the next visit.

Role Play #2: A 25-year-old mother with a history of a pain pill addiction, now being managed with methadone. She brings her 1-week-old baby in for a checkup. He has been fussy at times but otherwise he has been well. He is on a weaning dose schedule of methadone because of withdrawal symptoms in the nursery.

Objective

Use normalization to help mother discuss guilt about child's condition.

Trainee	Hello, Mrs. Moore
Mother	Please call me Heather.
Trainee	Heather, I'm Bill Cooper, a pediatric resident. Please call me Bill. So, Travis is here for a one week checkup. How is he doing?
Mother	Okay, but he is a bit fussy.
Trainee	Tell me more about the fussiness.
Mother	He just gets fussy. I don't think he is hungry.
Trainee	Lots of parents of babies who cry wonder if they caused the crying somehow by what they are doing or not doing. Is that true for you?
Mother	I do wonder if it is the methadone.
Trainee	So you think using methadone has caused your baby to be fussy?
Mother	I think he may be withdrawing. I feel pretty bad about it.
Trainee	Tell me why you are thinking he is withdrawing.

Feedback

Faculty	Good. Let's stop here. (*to trainee*) What do you think you did well in the interview?
Trainee	I thought I was nonjudgmental. I used normalization to ask her about her feelings.
Mother	I felt you cared about my feelings by the tone of your voice.
Faculty	I agree. Do you have any options?
Mother	I thought it was a little quick. I did not feel ready to talk to you about my guilt.
Faculty	(*to trainee*) What do you think?
Trainee	I agree.
Faculty	Let's do it again. This time you might set the stage by getting to know the mother first. You could ask her for her personal story.
Trainee	Okay.

Replay

Trainee	Heather, I see that Travis is here for his 1-week checkup. Before we get started on that, I'd like to hear about you as a person. I find it important to get to know families before getting started with medical issues.
Mother	I'm 25. Travis is my first baby. I used to work as a cashier. I've not worked since last year.
Trainee	Tell me more about yourself.
Mother	I think I am generally a nice person.
Trainee	This is your first baby. You are a nice person. Say more.
Mother	Well, I want to be a good mother. It means everything to me. I come from a large family and we always had children around. I have babysat since I was 12-years-old.
Trainee	You are very committed to being a good mother for Travis.
Mother	Yes. I do worry about him being on methadone.
Trainee	How do you think it is going so far?
Mother	Well, he gets fussy, and I can't calm him sometimes.
Trainee	What do you think might be causing it?
Mother	I don't know. I just want it to stop.
Trainee	Of course. Lots of parents of babies who cry wonder if they caused the crying somehow by what they did or didn't do. Is that true for you?
Mother	Yes. I think it might be the methadone he is on. It is my fault.

(continued)

Trainee	Are you thinking your baby is withdrawing?
Mother	Yes. And, I feel awful about it.
Trainee	That he is in pain as a result of your use of methadone?
Mother	Yes.

Feedback

Faculty	Okay. Good job. (*to mother*) Did you notice any difference this time?
Mother	Yes. I felt comfortable with him and ready to talk.
Faculty	What did the interviewer do to help you feel comfortable talking this time?
Mother	He took his time and got to know me a little first.
Faculty	Will you tell him directly?
Mother	You took your time and got to know me first. You had a soft voice and did not sound judgmental. And, you said that lots of parents of crying babies have guilty feelings—that I was not the only person in this position. It helped me calm myself a little. Of course, I still feel regret.
Faculty	Sure. One final comment… when the mother said she felt awful, I might have acknowledged her pain with a empathic statement, such as, "I imagine it is very painful to think you caused your baby to suffer."

Obstacles to Teaching Accuracy

1. Interviewer jumps to conclusions.
2. Interviewer believes that patients are either good or bad historians.
3. Interviewer lacks self-awareness during the interview.

Strategies

1. Educate trainees that jumping to conclusions is the leading type of diagnostic error made by clinicians.
2. Demonstrate to trainees how the interview is a dynamic process in which each person impacts the other. One way to accomplish this is for the trainee to experience the patient role, while the clinician uses different interviewing styles.
3. As part of role play supervision, ask trainees: what are you experiencing?

Accuracy

Is the interviewer obtaining the information he or she is trying to obtain?

Three aspects of the clinician–patient relationship are crucial to achieving this core function of the medical interview:

1. How does the **style of the interviewer** influence the process of obtaining a full and accurate history? Intuitively, one might guess that it has a major impact. The scientific evidence supports that view.
2. How can an interviewer effectively deal with patients who have characteristics, such as **vagueness,** that block the process of obtaining a full and accurate history? Specific interviewing techniques are often needed for these patients.
3. What approach is best when dealing with **sensitive** health issues, so that patients do not withhold vital information from the clinician? These topics include suicidality, sex, substance abuse, and violence to others.

Clinician Interviewing Style

Studies done over the last three decades have identified a number of physician interviewing characteristics that lead to incomplete databases. Among them are the following:

1. Omitting personal or psychosocial data, simply by not asking for it [1]. Of course, a clinician would not omit psychosocial data if he or she thought it was important. That is the problem. Some clinicians mistakenly believe it is not important. A clinician has an incomplete database when he or she does not uncover that an adolescent with chest pain has an uncle who recently died of a myocardial infarction.
2. Using high-control interviews. Instead of starting the interview with an invitation for the patient to tell his or her story, the clinician asks a series of questions that the patient must answer "yes" or "no." Some clinicians begin with one open-ended question before resorting to this high-control style, a style that is likely to leave out information. This information can be critical to accurate medical diagnosis [1–3]. Platt and McMath originally described this misguided attempt to save time back in 1979, and it is still commonly seen in 2013. A more effective approach is to invite the patient to fully tell his or her story, and then using a combination of focused and open-ended questions to fill in the details.
3. Not allowing the patient to list all of his problems and concerns early in the visit. Many patients, especially older ones, have multiple problems, which need to be prioritized in terms of clinical importance and time available. Problems not identified early are either brought up near the end of the visit, when time is limited, or the problem is not brought up at all [4, 5].
4. Insufficient inquiry into the details of the patient's symptoms. Patients provide the illness narrative. The clinician must ask focused questions to obtain the specific

facts not mentioned by the patient, but needed for accurate diagnosis [6]. It would certainly be a rare patient who knows and spontaneously describes all the important historical details.

5. Not summarizing the patient's story, *Let me see if I have this right …*, and asking the patient for corrections. Clinicians who do not check the accuracy of the history are susceptible to listening errors. The summarizing technique is modeled after the airline industry, and is standard in any high-risk profession. Medical data are crucial to health outcomes. It is important that the clinician get the history right [6].

These styles of interviewing take on added importance with recent studies showing the most common diagnostic error physicians make is premature closure (i.e., jumping to conclusions) [7, 8].

Patients Who Are Vague

The most important part of the database is the history of present illness. Ideally, the patient stays on track while describing his or her illness story in a chronological manner, providing the clinician with the detailed information needed to make a correct diagnosis. In reality, most patients do not do this because something gets in the way. The conversational style of the patient is one of the more common blocks encountered in primary care. Some patients simply give vague responses. Any number of conditions can result in a vague patient. Most commonly, it is secondary to one of the following: anxiety, a personality style, a unique set of beliefs by the patient regarding how symptoms and events are related, or it signifies a true cognitive impairment [9]. Every effort to find the cause and respond effectively should be made so that a solid database is obtained. The first cause to consider is a possible cognitive impairment, since that will change the direction of the interview.

Cognitive Deficit

Cognitive impairments, due to dementia, delirium, and structural brain conditions (e.g., stroke), are frequent in primary care [6]. It is common for the busy clinician to miss or underestimate the degree of cognitive impairment because patients frequently compensate for their deficits [6]. Some impaired patients are easy to engage, while others are agitated, hostile, or withdrawn [6]. Often, they are frightened. They provide histories full of irrelevant, incomplete, and illogical statements.

Once a clinician suspects a cognitive deficit, it is essential for the clinician to evaluate the patient's ability to provide an accurate history. Typically, the clinician has gotten a sense of the patient's cognitive impairment from the clinical presentation (e.g., adult daughter drove the patient to the appointment; disheveled appearance) and the way he or she answers basic questions requiring memory (e.g., *What was the date of your recent operation?*) [9]. However, a standard mental status exam, such as the Mini Mental Status Exam, should be performed to obtain a fuller picture [10]. A transition statement smoothly guides the patient into this area: *Many patients with the type of medical problems you have notice changes in their memory. I would like to ask you a few questions to check that out.*

If the Mini Mental Status Exam results show a cognitive impairment, the clinician will need to interview third-party sources to obtain a full and accurate history. When talking with cognitively impaired patients, it is helpful to keep in mind that they are likely frightened and may not understand the verbal concepts being discussed. Therefore, empathic **nonverbal communication**, such as a soft, even voice and a relaxed forward-leaning body posture, helps support verbalizations such as: *I imagine that this is frightening* [6].

Vagueness

For a vague patient without a cognitive impairment, it is important to let the patient talk and listen attentively for the initial 3–5 min, just as with a wandering patient. (See Chap. 7 for a discussion of structuring wandering patients.) He or she has the same need to be heard as anyone else. Again, clinician frustration will only increase vagueness and thereby compromise the accuracy and completeness of the data. For a vague patient who tries to talk about a host of problems all at once, it can be helpful to state: *Let's take this one problem at a time. What do you think is your main concern?*

Increasing Precision with Vague Patients

Vague patients have difficulty describing a symptom. Certain symptoms, such as dizziness, drowsiness, and lack of energy, can be hard to describe for any patient. Vague patients have trouble being specific and clear about almost any symptom. Clarifying techniques for decreasing vagueness can be effective [9].

Patient	I feel ill.
Clinician	Tell me what you mean by "ill."
Patient	I just don't feel right. I've got the flu.
Clinician	Tell me more about the flu.
Patient	My muscles hurt.

This clinician simply asked the patient to be more precise (*Tell me what you mean by ill/flu*) A second specific technique is often necessary with these patients. The clinician offers a **menu of options** from which to choose, such as: *By the flu, do* *you mean cough, fever, and muscle aches, or do you mean nausea, vomiting and diarrhea, or something else?* [9]. The risk of offering a menu of options is that the patient may choose one that does not accurately reflect the patient's experience.

Recall Errors

Even when patients are not vague and do not ramble, the symptoms reported to the clinician may not be accurate because of error in recall. Recall of symptoms can be affected by the one's emotional state (e.g., anxiety, depression), by the remoteness in time of the events described, and a host of other factors [11]. Two general interviewing techniques may help accurate recall of symptoms:

1. Use anchor points—a memorable date, such as a birthday party or holiday that occurred during the period in question [12].
2. Ask the patient to recall the sequence of events, starting with the most recent event and moving backward in time, since this increases recall [13].

Interviewing Tools for Sensitive Issues

An important task of providing comprehensive health care involves asking patients about health risk behaviors that they may be reluctant to share because of feelings of guilt, shame, or thoughts of inadequacy. These topics include sexual behaviors, violence toward others, suicidal thoughts and behaviors, and substance abuse. Patients can also be sensitive about feelings experienced as part of everyday life, for which they judge themselves negatively. For example, a parent may feel resentful or irritated with a newborn's crying, and not share those feelings with the clinician because of shame. If the parent discussed this with the clinician, he or she might learn it is common to have such feelings, and find healthy ways of dealing with those feelings. In this instance and in similar instances, it is important for the clinician to make it emotionally safe for the patient to talk. Unconditional, positive regard and a nonjudgmental stance help patients trust that it is safe to talk. That may not be enough to encourage a patient to discuss a sensitive topic. Clinicians often need to use specific interviewing techniques to smoothly elicit sensitive material. Shawn Shea has identified normalization, gentle assumption, denial of the specific, and behavioral incident as four examples of such tools [14].

Normalization

With normalization, a question or statement is phrased so that the patient appreciates that his or her feelings, thoughts, and behaviors are typical of other human beings. This technique can help diminish the patient's self-judgment and shame, inviting him or her to share hidden feelings, thoughts, and behaviors [14].

| Clinician | Lots of people who have the type of depression you are experiencing right now have thoughts of ending their life, of suicide. Is that true for you? |
| Patient | I've thought it would be okay if I didn't wake up in the morning. But I wouldn't kill myself. |

Gentle Assumption

The technique of gentle assumption assumes a particular behavior or thought (e.g., suicidal ideation, marijuana use) is occurring by the manner in which the question is framed. The clinician implies that the behavior is expected. This can act to decrease shame and make it feel safe for the patient to reveal sensitive information [14].

Clinician	Have you had thoughts of killing yourself?
Patient	Not really. (*implies he/she has had thoughts*)
Clinician	What thoughts have you had? (*gentle assumption*)
Patient	Well, …

Gentle assumption could act as a leading question for a patient trying to please the physician. Therefore, **it should never be used when asking about childhood physical or sexual abuse,** since false memories could be reported [14].

Denial of the Specific

Instead of making open-ended, general inquires, the clinician asks the patient one or more specific questions. This forces the patient to deny specific acts, which can be difficult for a patient to do [14]. Denial of the specific can be particularly helpful when asking about substance abuse or when exploring certain aspects of suicidal ideation [14, 15].

Clinician	Have you been using alcohol or drugs recently?
Patient	I drink 2–3 beers occasionally.
Clinician	How about marijuana?
Patient	I might use once a day, sometimes twice.
Clinician	What's the amount you use in a typical week?
Patient	Probably 10–15 joints.
Clinician	Do you use speed or methamphetamine?
Patient	No, not at all.
Clinician	How about Cocaine?

Behavioral Incident

Psychiatrist Gerald Pascal observed marked disparities between hospitalized patients' reports of their childhood experiences and the actual happenings. When Pascal asked them to describe the quality of their childhood relationships, patients often replied "fine." Yet, during the hospitalization, they would describe childhood stories of neglect and harsh treatment. He coined the term **behavioral incident** to signify the act of uncovering facts of the story, versus receiving patient opinion. The clinician obtains a chronological history of concrete, specific behaviors, carefully tracking with the patient [16]. Behavioral incidents can be implemented as an interviewing technique for both sensitive topics and routine medical problems. The only drawback to employing a behavioral incident is the amount of time expended [14]. Therefore, the clinician must choose when it would be important to obtain specific, concrete details.

Assessing suicidal thought and behaviors is one of the important times to use a behavioral incident.

Clinician	David, tell me about what happened yesterday when your mother called you to come into the house.
Patient	I got mad.
Clinician	And then what happened?
Patient	I said I wasn't going to come inside.
Clinician	What happened next?
Patient	Mom said, "Yes you are."
Clinician	Then?
Patient	I said, "No I'm not." I started to run.
Clinician	What were you thinking as you ran?
Patient	I'm going to get away from her.
Clinician	And then what did you do?
Patient	I ran across the street.
Clinician	What were you thinking was going to happen to you?
Patient	I thought I might get hit by a car.
Clinician	Did you want to get hit by a car?
Patient	No. I just wanted to get away. [17]

Key Points

1. Clinicians can increase accuracy by allowing the patient the space to tell his or her story and then using a combination of focused and open-ended questions to fill in the details needed for an accurate diagnosis.
2. Consider the possibility of a cognitive impairment in patients who ramble or are vague.

3. It is important for clinicians to gain as much precision as possible when patients use vague descriptors.
4. Specific validity techniques, such as normalization and behavioral incidents, increase accuracy with sensitive and critical issues, such as suicide assessments.

References

1. Platt FW, McMath JC. Clinical hypocompetence: the interview. Ann Intern Med. 1979;91:898–902.
2. Cox A, Rutter M, Holbrook D. Psychiatric interviewing techniques. V. Experimental study: eliciting factual information. Br J Psychiatry. 1981;139:29–37.
3. Linfors EW, Neelon FA. Interrogation and interview: strategies for obtaining clinical data. J R Coll Gen Pract. 1981;31:426–8.
4. Beckman HB, Frankel RM. The effect of physician behavior on the collection of data. Ann Intern Med. 1984;101:692–6.
5. Marvel KM, Epstein RM, Flowers K, Beckman HB. Soliciting the patient's agenda: have we improved? JAMA. 1999;281:283–7.
6. Platt FW, Gordon GH. Field guide to the difficult patient interview. 2nd ed. Philadelphia, PA: Lippincott Williams and Wilkins; 2004.
7. Graber ML, Franklin N, Gordon R. Diagnostic error in internal medicine. Arch Intern Med. 2005;165:1493–9.
8. Croskerry P. Achieving quality in clinical decision making: cognitive strategies and detection of bias. Acad Emerg Med. 2002;9:1184–204.
9. Coulehan JL, Block MR. The medical interview: mastering skills for clinical practice. 5th ed. Philadelphia, PA: F. A Davis; 2006.
10. Folstein MF, Folstein SE, McHugh PR. "Mini-mental state." A practical method for grading the cognitive state of patients for the clinician. J Psychiatr Res. 1975;12:189–98.
11. Barsky AJ. Forgetting, fabricating and telescoping: the instability of the medical history. Arch Intern Med. 2002;162:981–4.
12. Loftus EF, Marburger W. Since the eruption of Mt. St. Helens, has anyone beaten you up? Improving the accuracy of retrospective reports with landmark events. Mem Cognit. 1983;11:114–20.
13. Loftus EF, Fathi D. Retrieving multiple autobiographical memories. Soc Cognit. 1985;3:280–95.
14. Shea SC. Psychiatric interviewing: the art of understanding: a practical guide for psychiatrists, psychologists, counselors, social workers, nurses and other health professionals. 2nd ed. Philadelphia, PA: WB Saunders; 1998.
15. Shea SC. The practical art of suicide assessment: a guide for mental health professionals and substance abuse counselors. Hoboken, NJ: Wiley; 2002.
16. Pascal G. The practical art of diagnostic interviews. Homewood, IL: Dow Jones-Irwin; 1983.
17. Binder J. Pediatric Interviewing: a practical relationship-based approach. New York, NY: Humana Press; 2010.

Chapter 9
History of Present Illness

"Your patient's symptoms are the gold of medical interviewing."

F. Platt and G. Gordon

Role Play

Prerequisite Interviewing Skills:

Role Play #1:   *Attending* and *listening, open-ended questioning, facilitating (echoing, silence), empathic summaries,* and *transition statements.*

Role Play #2:   *Focused questioning,* clarifying, *weaving opened-ended,* closed-ended *questioning,* and *staying in one region until completion.*

   Role Play #1:   44-year-old woman presents with urinary frequency.

Objectives

1. Invite the patient to tell her illness narrative.
2. Use at least two empathic summaries before transitioning to doctor-type questions.

Trainee	Mrs. Brown, tell me the reason for the visit today.
Patient	I'm urinating a lot, but I don't feel sick.
Trainee	Anything else?
Patient	No, that's it.
Trainee	Tell me about the urinary frequency.
Patient	I started urinating frequently yesterday afternoon. I go almost every hour.
Trainee	Are you urinating small or large amounts?

(continued)

The online version of this chapter (doi:10.1007/978-1-4614-7224-7_9) contains supplementary material, which is available to authorized users.

J. Binder, *Primary Care Interviewing: Learning Through Role Play*,
DOI 10.1007/978-1-4614-7224-7_9, © Springer Science+Business Media New York 2013

| Patient | Small amounts. |
| Trainee | Does it burn? |

Time Out

Faculty	(*gives "time out" signal*) Let me stop you for a second. These are good questions, just too soon. It is better to ask them after the patient gets a chance to tell her narrative.
Trainee	I can see I've already moved to the doctor questions.
Faculty	Right. One way you could avoid that trap is first to get the patient on track, then use summaries to support the patient telling her story. You might get her on track with a statement like, "Tell me everything about your urine, the pressure and anything else about your illness. Start at the beginning and walk me through it."
Trainee	Okay.

Replay

Trainee	Mrs. Brown, what brings you in today?
Patient	I've been urinating a lot. I also feel some pressure in my bottom.
Trainee	Anything else?
Patient	No, that's it.
Trainee	Tell me all about your illness—frequent urination and the pressure. Start at the beginning and walk me through it.
Patient	It started yesterday. I urinated every 1–2 hours during the night. I didn't sleep very well. It's no better today and now I also feel a pressure.
Trainee	Let me see if I have it so far. You started urinating frequently yesterday and were up much of the night. Today you feel a pressure in your bottom? (*patient nods*) Tell me more.
Faculty	(*interrupts*) That gentle command at the end of your summary is an excellent way to keep the patient on track. Back to you, Mrs. Brown.
Patient	Well, the pressure when I urinate is painful. And, I don't feel so good. I thought I might have another UTI—like I had a few years ago—but the urine looks totally clear. I thought something might be pressing on my bladder.

(continued)

Trainee	So you don't feel so good and feel pressure with urination. You thought it might be another UTI. However, your urine looks clear. You wonder if something is pressing on your bladder. Do you feel anxiety about that?
Patient	Not really.
Trainee	Tell me more about your illness.
Patient	I don't have any fever. That's about it.
Trainee	Uh-huh. I'd like to shift to doctor-type questions to get a fuller picture of your illness.
Patient	Okay.

Feedback

Faculty	Let's stop. Nice job. You got a contract for the session. I like the way you set the patient up to tell her narrative. You listened without interrupting. You used 2 empathic summaries and invited her to say more. You smoothly transitioned to doctor-type questions.

Demonstration to trainees

The faculty member models the interviewing skills required for the second role play before the trainee attempts Role Play #2.

Role Play #2: A 29-year-old woman presents with dysuria and cloudy urine.

Objectives

1. Fully assess the seven dimensions of the symptoms, finishing one dimension before moving on to the next.
2. Use open-ended questions to enter each new region and whenever the patient gives an affirmative response to an inquiry.

Trainee	I'd like to ask you some doctor-type questions to better understand your illness.
Patient	Okay.
Trainee	You mentioned that urinating became painful two days ago. Tell me what it feels like.
Patient	It burns whenever I urinate.
Trainee	How severe is it?

(continued)

Patient	It definitely burns.
Trainee	Did it start gradually or come on all of a sudden?
Patient	It came on rather suddenly. I was on a hike at the time.
Trainee	Have you noticed other symptoms?
Patient	Well, the cloudy urine, like I told you. I don't feel good and have a fever today.
Trainee	Let me see if I have everything so far. You have noticed burning when you urinate, starting two days ago. Today you don't feel good and think you might have a fever. You have also noticed that your urine is cloudy. Anything else?
Patient	I had chills earlier this morning.
Trainee	Do you any other symptoms?
Patient	No, that's it.
Trainee	Stop me if you have had any of the following: frequent urination, urgency, pain
Patient	(interrupts) Yes, I go every couple of hours.
Trainee	Is the amount less than usual or more than usual?
Patient	It's less.
Trainee	When you feel the urge to urinate, do you have to go immediately?
Patient	Maybe a little.
Trainee	And, do you ever void involuntarily?
Patient	No.
Trainee	So let me summarize once again. You have had burning when you urinate for 2 days and a cloudy urine. You are urinating small amounts and feel urgency. Currently, you have fever and don't feel well.
Patient	Yes.
Trainee	Do you have any pain in your lower back or flank?
Patient	My left lower back has been hurting.
Trainee	Tell me more about it.
Patient	I thought I might have injured my back. It feels achy.
Trainee	When did the pain start?
Patient	Yesterday afternoon.
Trainee	Does it come and go or is it there all the time?
Patient	It's constant.
Trainee	How severe?
Patient	Pretty bad.
Trainee	Let me see if I have everything so far. You started with frequent and painful urination 2 days ago. Now you have fever, chills, pain in your left lower back and don't feel well. Is that right?
Patient	Yes.
Trainee	Have you had any vaginal discharge?
Patient	No.
Trainee	Have you noticed any other effects on your general health besides the fever, chills, and not feeling well?

(continued)

Patient	I don't think so.
Trainee	How about your appetite?
Patient	It's poor. I am drinking okay.
Trainee	Have you changed anything as far as your activities?
Patient	I've stayed in bed today.
Trainee	Have you tried anything, like medication, to feel better?
Patient	Tylenol. It didn't help.

Feedback

Faculty	Let's stop. You did a nice job of fulfilling the two objectives of the role play. You carved out all the descriptors of the dysuria and then did the same with the flank pain. Of course, there was overlap in terms of associated symptoms. You also used open-ended questions to enter each region and you weaved them in when you could. I particularly like your use of empathic summaries. You used three of them. That is likely to increase your accuracy and rapport.

Role Play: Front to Back (1&2)

Faculty	I believe you are ready to do the two role plays front to back. This time you will start at the very beginning and go all the way through. Do you feel ready?
Trainee	Sure.

Obstacles to Teaching History of Present Illness

1. Interviewer believes that a series of closed-ended questions saves time. Sometimes, a clinician will ask one or two open-ended questions before resorting to closed-ended questioning.
2. Interviewer avoids empathic summaries because of a belief that they are unnecessary or a fear that patients will experience them as repetitive and mechanical.
3. Interviewer is careless about obtaining the details of the seven descriptors.

Strategies

1. Educate trainees regarding the connection between an exclusively closed-ended questioning style and a deficient database.
2. Educate trainees on the empirical studies showing a connection between open-ended inquiries and accurate data collection (see Chap. 8).
3. Invite trainees to experiment with the use of empathic summaries, and observe patient response.
4. Emphasize the importance of obtaining a full and accurate history in order to avoid jumping to conclusions.

History of Present Illness

Uncovering a hidden diagnosis is one of the most satisfying experiences in medicine. The ability of the diagnostician to make the right diagnosis is, in large measure, dependent on his or her ability to obtain a full and accurate history. Premature closure is a common cause of misdiagnoses [1]. Occasionally, a physician will recognize a classic pattern of symptoms that is highly suggestive of one diagnosis (e.g., chronic honking cough that disappears with sleep and the diagnosis of a psychogenic cough). Even less often, the physician might discover a single question that clearly discriminates conditions (e.g., eye opening versus eyes closed during an ictal event possesses a high discriminatory power for epileptic versus non-epileptic seizures, when accurately ascertained [2]). Much more often, clinical practice requires careful, methodical reasoning utilizing the principles of epidemiology and clinical medicine to formulate a solid differential diagnosis.

Myth: A correct diagnosis is frequently made as the result of a clever hunch.

In Chap. 8, we reviewed strong evidence that a full and accurate history is dependent on <u>both</u> open-ended and focused questions. The history of present illness must be structured in a way that makes that possible. The following strategy is one way for the clinician and patient to build the history collaboratively.

Preliminary Work

The *history of present illness*[1] begins during the opening phase with an invitation to the patient to tell his or her illness story. This occurs immediately after the personal story has been narrated and a contract for the session made (see Chaps. 1 and 2). Sometimes preliminary work must be done to help the patient get on track to tell his or her illness story [4, 5]. A patient might not be clear when naming the symptom.

---

[1]The proposed plan for building the hpi together is adapted from Lin et al. [3].

For example, the patient describes his or her symptoms as: *I have no energy*. Another patient may use clear terminology, but focus on secondary data, such as previous diagnoses and treatments. Neither of these patients is providing the primary symptom data needed by the clinician to make a good diagnosis. The clinician can help these patients get on track with structuring techniques:

1. Clarification of patient's concern, translating it into a symptom [6].

Clinician	Tell me what you mean when you say you have no energy.
Patient	I don't have energy to do things I used to do.
Clinician	Do you mean you are tired and not sleeping well, or that your motivation to do activities, such as chores, is low, or do you mean you get short of breath with exertion, or maybe something else?

2. Tell the patient what is needed [4].

Clinician	I would like to first understand your symptoms—burning with urination, abdominal pain, fever—that type of thing. This will help me get a better picture of your illness. We'll come back to the previous tests and treatments you have had. Is that okay?
Patient	Sure.

Secondary Data

Some clinicians do gather secondary (nonsymptom) data first, especially with patients who have had extensive medical evaluations and treatment in the past. It is important that these clinicians then return and obtain symptom data. Symptoms can be viewed as primary data—facts known to the patient. The nonsymptom data tend to be more a matter of hearsay, thus not really known to the patient. If one relies on the secondary data, past mistakes in diagnoses get perpetuated.

Primary Data

Once any preliminary work is completed, the clinician gives an invitation for the patient to tell his or her story: *So, tell me about the burning, abdominal pain and fever and everything else about your illness. Start at the beginning and walk me through it.* It is helpful to demonstrate to trainees the actual words to say. Their natural tendency is to jump right in with focused questions (e.g., *Where does it hurt?*) The trainees are instructed to "bite your tongue" rather than give in to the urge to ask a focused question early on in the interview. After 1–2 min, the trainee responds to the patient's narrative with an empathic summary [3]: *Let me see if I have this so far. You have had burning when you urinate for 2 days, fever and chills beginning this morning, and pain in your flank area. You are concerned you have another kidney infection. Is that right?* At the conclusion of the first empathic summary, the trainee is strongly encouraged to use another gentle command to help the patient stay on track telling his or her story: *Tell me more about your illness.* Again, the trainee avoids focused questions [3]. Once the patient's story begins to taper off, perhaps after two or three empathic summaries, the trainee uses a transition statement to guide the interview to focused questions.

Patient	I don't have any appetite.
Clinician	Let me see if I have this so far.... (*empathic summary*) Is this right? (*patient nods*) I would like to shift now and ask you some doctor-type questions [4].

Focused Questions

Symptoms have seven classic descriptors (chronology, location, quality, quantity, associated symptoms, setting, and transforming factors) [7]. Smith et al. suggest carefully assessing the descriptors of each primary symptom, which can be done simultaneously for symptoms grouped chronologically. This is followed by an inquiry into relevant nonsymptom data [6]. A careful approach is warranted, given evidence that both medical students and practicing physicians commonly miss important details [8, 9]. I want to mark the importance of being precise with a brief story a cardiologist told me this week (Table 9.1).

A 38 yr. old man presented with non-exertional chest discomfort. FH was positive for sudden death in the PGF. A nuclear stress 8 months prior had been negative. The cardiologist reassured the patient and prescribed NSAIDS. He also asked the patient to keep a 2-week log of the chest discomfort. The patient called back and stated he had two episodes of central chest pressure with jogging. A coronary CT scan revealed an anomalous left coronary artery from the right aortic cusp, which has an association with sudden death. Surgery was successfully performed. **Precision does matter.**

The following is a thumbnail sketch of the seven descriptors. Beginning interviewers are more likely to obtain a complete database if they follow the same order of asking about symptom descriptors each time, so they don't leave out any dimensions. The mnemonic **OPQQRST (Onset and chronology, Position and radiation, Quality, Quantification, Related symptoms, Setting, and Transforming (aggravating/ alleviating) factors** is a helpful guide for students [6]. Chronology forms the framework for the other descriptors (Table 9.2).

Table 9.1 Structure—HPI

1. Invite the patient to tell the story of his or her illness immediately after the personal story and contracting are completed (*Tell me about the urinary frequency and fever. Start at the beginning and walk me through it*)
2. Make an empathic summary every 1–2 min, followed by silence and then another gentle command. Avoid focused questions at this point (*Tell me more*)
3. Use a transition statement when the patient's story is winding down (*I'd like to ask you some doctor-type questions*)
4. Ask about the seven descriptors of the symptoms
   - Use an open-to-closed questioning approach
   - Weave in a gentle command when a patient responds "yes" to a focused question
   - Continue to use empathic summaries every 1–2 min
5. Obtain the seven descriptors for the other main symptoms concurrently or sequentially
6. Ask about relevant nonsymptom data from the PMH, SH, and FH, including previous diagnoses, testing, and treatment

Table 9.2 The seven descriptors of symptoms (OPQQRST)

1. **O**nset and chronology
   When did it begin? How long does it last? How often does it happen?
   (a) Time of onset of symptom and intervals between recurrences
   (b) Duration of symptoms
   (c) Periodicity and frequency of symptom
   (d) Time course of symptom
      (i) Short-term
      (ii) Long-term
2. **P**osition and radiation
   Where is it located? Does it travel anywhere?
   (a) Precise location
3. **Q**uality
   What is it like?
   (a) Usual descriptors
   (b) Unusual descriptors
4. **Q**uantification
   How bad is it? For pain: *On a scale of 1 to 10, with 1 being no pain and 10 being the worst pain you can imagine, like surgery without anesthesia, what number would you give your pain?*
   (a) Type of onset
   (b) Intensity or severity
   (c) Impairment or disability
   (d) Numeric description
      (i) Number of events
      (ii) Size
      (iii) Volume
5. **R**elated symptoms
   Have you noticed anything else that occurs with it?

(continued)

Table 9.2 (continued)

6. Setting (circumstances that contribute to or precipitate the symptom)
   (a) Environmental factors
   (b) Social factors
   (c) Activity
   (d) Emotions
7. Transforming factors
   What brings it on? What makes it better? What makes it worsen
   (a) Precipitating and aggravating factors
   (b) Relieving factors

Copied with permission from Smith's Patient-Centered Interviewing: an Evidence-Based Method (2012) by Fortin, Dwamena, Frankel, and Smith

Onset and Chronology

Establish the time of onset, duration, intervals, and course using calendar time [7]. If the patient can use specific landmarks like a birthday or holiday, confidence in the accuracy of the timeline is increased. All time intervals need to be accounted. If the symptoms are episodic, a recent, specific example is examined, the long-term course is defined, and individual episodes are placed on a timeline. Patients are asked: *Then what happened*? Obtaining all relevant details helps the interviewer understand the big picture [7]. It is helpful to know why the patient or family decided to come at this time. *Have the symptoms persisted too long or increased in severity? Did they begin to worry?*

Position and Radiation

An attempt to obtain a precise description is made. An area of pain may be small or large, may be superficial or deep, or may radiate or not. Patients can be asked to point to their pain. *Is the pain on the surface or deep? Does it move anywhere?* The description of the location and radiation can help the clinician formulate hypotheses [7]. For example, colicky, severe pain in the flank suggests urinary obstruction secondary to a renal calculus.

Quality

Quality is ascertained by asking what the symptom feels like [7]. Most patients are eager to describe the qualities of the symptom and may use highly metaphorical language. Sometimes this is helpful diagnostically, as with the sudden onset of tearing chest pain in aortic dissection (quality and quantity) [10]. Other times, the quality does not help us diagnostically. For example, common descriptors of pain may help us understand a patient's experience, but not point toward a specific diagnosis [4]. If the patient does not describe the symptom, one strategy is to list choices [6]: *Is the pain dull, achy, sharp, crushing?* The problem with that strategy is that a patient may attempt to fit his or her symptoms into one of the categories, instead of describing the symptom in his or her own terms. Sometimes a patient who has difficulty describing a symptom will respond to being asked a second time: *How would you describe the pain?*

Quantification

A number of features must be considered in this category: type of onset (sudden, gradual, etc.), intensity or severity, functional impairment, and numerical descriptors (number of events, size, volume, etc.) [6]. Functional impairment is an important measure of severity. A useful way to assess functional impairment is to ask the patient to describe his or her activities on a specific recent day. This is likely to be more accurate than asking about activities on a typical day [7].

Related Symptoms

Clinical illnesses commonly present with a **group of symptoms** that are related. Associated or related symptoms stem from both the local and generalized effects of the disease. Different combinations of symptoms have diagnostic significance [6]. Dysuria, frequency, and hematuria (local symptoms) are commonly seen together in patients with a urinary tract infection. General effects include fever, chills, a change in activity, etc. Both types of associated symptoms must be systematically assessed [6].

A patient presenting with dysuria would need to be asked about other symptoms from the body system that appears to be involved, the urinary system—frequency, urgency, loss of control of urine, bloody or cloudy urine, and flank pain. Then, the patient should be asked about any other body system that could reasonably cause the symptom; in this case, the genital system. Men would be asked about urethral discharge; women would be asked about vaginal discharge and pain with sexual intercourse. In addition, the clinician asks about secondary **general** symptoms (activity level, appetite, affect, fever, chills, pain, and change in weight). They are important indicators of the severity of the illness [6].

Clinician	Tell me what effect the illness has had on your general health.
Patient	I'm not sure.
Clinician	Stop me if you have had any of the following general symptoms: change in activity, appetite, weight, mood, any fever and chills...
Patient	Only my appetite.
Clinician	What change have you noticed?

Setting

Exploring what the patient was doing and where he or she was as the symptoms developed can help characterize a symptom, as well as give a window into the life of the patient. *Tell me what you were doing and where you were at the time you became ill?* Often, this information is obtained during the patient's initial narrative. At times, the clinician must specifically ask about recent events such as travel [7].

Transforming (Aggravating/Alleviating) Factors

A symptom can be influenced by activities such as eating, exercising, and sleeping. The patient is asked about any factors that appear to help or worsen the condition [7].

Tell me anything that seems to aggravate or bring out the pain. If the patient found that hard to answer, a clinician might try: *Tell me what you have found you have to avoid, so the pain doesn't reappear or get worse?*

Similarly, if a patient is unable to say what lessens a symptom, it may be helpful to ask: *What do you find yourself doing after you get this symptom?*

Conversational Style

Once the middle phase of the interview has been initiated, the clinician can easily fall into a pattern of asking a series of closed-ended questions, a style that disengages many patients. The following techniques foster a conversational feeling and avoid a string of yes/no answers [3]:

1. Use a gentle command when entering each new descriptor region. *Tell me what other symptoms you have noticed.* (Details not mentioned by the patient are obtained with focused questioning: *Stop me if you have had any of the following symptoms: frequent urination, urge to urinate, blood in the urine, loss of control of your urine, flank pain…*)
2. **Weave** in a gentle command whenever the patient responds yes to a focused inquiry [4].

Patient	Yes.
Clinician	Yes to which one?
Patient	Blood in the urine.
Clinician	Tell me about it. (*weaving in an open-ended inquiry*)

3. Continue to summarize during this phase of the interview [3]. *Let me see if I have everything so far....*

The art of this phase of the interview is being able to guide the interview to the necessary details without disengaging the patient. As we noted in Chap. 7, **it is important, in terms of time efficiency and the completeness of the database, to fully assess one region at a time.** If the clinician does leave a content region to explore a patient's theory of illness or respond to a patient's emotions, he or she simply guides the interview back to the same content area once the excursion is completed.

Clinical Context

An inductive method of clinical reasoning can be time consuming. Trainees are dependent on it; experienced diagnosticians are not. Seasoned clinicians develop theories very early, incorporating further data to substantiate or dismiss their initial hypothesis [11]. They move from the general to the specific to avoid the hazard of leaving out important, alternative diagnoses. Because of their clinical experiences and knowledge, they ask questions that differentiate conditions, without necessarily inquiring about every detail a trainee would obtain [12]. For example, if a patient has recurrent headaches for 2 years with features of tension headaches, the clinician might scan the neurological review of symptoms with only a few questions (e.g., visual changes, motor weakness, vomiting) to ensure he or she is not missing a more serious diagnosis. Conversely, if a child presented with a progressive headache for a month, he or she would fully scan associated neurological symptoms because of the greater possibility of a central nervous system lesion and/or increased intracranial pressure.

The context for a symptom or group of symptoms includes secondary data. The clinician completes the database by inquiring about previous diagnoses, medications, hospitalizations, as well as any relevant data from the past medical history, social, family, and travel history [6]. He or she integrates the above information with known epidemiological factors, such as gender, age, and season of the year to formulate a differential diagnosis. For example, it would be important for a clinician evaluating a young child with recurrent headaches—as in the above scenario—to be knowledgeable that migraine headaches do occur in young children with many of the same features as in adults [13]. Children with migraines have a positive family history of migraine headaches, feel sick, and are quiet [13]. A good diagnostician must learn the sensitivity and specificity of the questions he or she asks, such as: *Does the child become quiet?* [14].

Key Points

1. Symptoms are the primary data.
2. Empathic summaries offer clinicians an effective tool for checking the accuracy of the data, while simultaneously allowing them to empathize with the patient.
3. Open-ended and focused questioning can be smoothly integrated, enhancing both engagement and data collection.
4. It is important to be careful during the history of present illness to consider alternative diagnoses, so as not to jump to conclusions (a common error).

References

1. Graber ML, Franklin N, Gordon R. Diagnostic errors in internal medicine. Arch Intern Med. 2005;165:1493–9.
2. Chung SS, Gerber P, Kirlin KA. Ictal eye closure is a reliable indicator for psychogenic non-epileptic seizures. Neurology. 2006;66:1730–1.
3. Lin CT, Platt FW, Hardee JT, Boyle D, Leslie B, Dwinnell B. The medical inquiry: invite, listen, summarize. J Clin Outcomes Manag. 2005;12:415–8.
4. Platt FW, Gordon GH. Field guide to the difficult patient interview. 2nd ed. Philadelphia, PA: Lippincott Williams and Wilkins; 2004.
5. Coulehan JC, Block MR. The medical interview in mastering skills for clinical practice. 5th ed. Philadelphia, PA: F.A. Davis; 2006.
6. Fortin A, Dwamena FC, Frankel RM, Smith RC. Smith's patient-centered interviewing: an evidence-based method. 3rd ed. New York, NY: McGraw Hill; 2012.
7. Morgan WL, Engel GL. The clinical approach to the patient. Philadelphia, PA: WB Saunders; 1969.
8. Roter DL, Hall JA. Physicians' interviewing styles and medical information obtained from patients. J Gen Intern Med. 1987;2:325–9.
9. Maquire GP, Rutter DR. History taking for medical students: deficiencies in performance. Lancet. 1976;2:556–8.
10. von Kodolitsch Y, Schwartz AG, Nienaber CA. Clinical prediction of acute aortic dissection. Arch Intern Med. 2000;160:2977–82.
11. Sackett DL, Haynes RB, Guyatt GH, Tugwell P. Clinical epidemiology: a basic science for clinical medicine. 2nd ed. Boston, MA: Little Brown; 1991.
12. Barrows HS, Norman GR, Neufield VR, Feightner JW. The clinical reasoning of randomly selected physicians in general medical practice. Clin Invest Med. 1982;5:49–55.
13. Gupta A, Cohen BH. Headaches in children. In: Kliegman RM, Greenbaum LA, Lye PS, editors. Practical strategies in pediatric diagnosis and therapy. 2nd ed. Philadelphia, PA: Elsevier Saunders; 2004.
14. Davis G, Henderson MC, Smetana GW. The evidence-based approach to clinical decision making. In: Tierney LM, Henderson MC, editors. The patient history: evidence-based approach. New York, NY: Large Medical Book I McGraw Hill; 2005.

Chapter 10
Concluding Phase

Role Play

Prerequisite interviewing skills for role-playing the closing phase: *listening*, *elicit feelings*, *empathic summary*, *third-party technique*, *uncover* *theory of illness* *(self-diagnosis)*, *provide information without jargon, know the condition and treatment,* and *restatement*.

Role Play: A 70-year-old man presents with recent signs of congestive heart failure (CHF). He had been previously well. Workup suggested cardiomyopathy of undetermined etiology. He is accompanied to the visit by his son, a nurse.

Objectives

1. Explain medical condition to the patient and family in chunks. No jargon.
2. Use restatement.

Trainee	Mr. Smith, I am glad you brought your son. I would like to discuss your diagnosis and how we can best treat it, today. Is that plan okay with you?
Patient	Yes.
Trainee	You have congestive heart failure. Your heart is not pumping well. The fluid in your body is backing up. Also, your heart is not getting as much blood as it should to the organs in your body. This has

(continued)

DOI 10.1007/978-1-4614-7224-7_10, © Springer Science+Business Media New York 2013

resulted in the shortness of breath with physical exertion, as well as the fatigue you have experienced. It is a common condition. In fact, it becomes more common with age. In your case, I think, that a virus may have affected your heart and caused it to stop pumping normally. It is important that we monitor your condition carefully, so that you receive appropriate treatment. You will need to weigh yourself daily. You will stay on the medicines that were started when you were here last time. In addition, diet will be important.

Son   I live nearby and can help out by checking on my dad's condition.

Trainee   That's great. We will set up an action plan. We will keep track of your weight, your breathing.

Faculty   Let me jump in here for a second. (*to trainee*) What are you experiencing?

Trainee   A little tension.

Faculty   Tension due to what?

Trainee   I feel there is a lot of information I need to get across to Mr. Smith and his son.

Faculty   I can appreciate that—there is a lot of information. It is important to get that information across in a way Mr. Smith can receive it. Would you be willing to do an experiment? You be Mr. Smith for a little bit and let yourself experience what it is like to get this information.

Trainee   Sure.

Faculty   Mr. Smith, you have congestive heart failure. Your heart has not actually failed, but it is not pumping well. It is not effectively pumping blood to the organs in your body. The result is that you have been tired and short of breath when you walk. It is a common condition. It becomes even more common with age. I think you developed this problem after a viral infection. I will monitor you closely so you can receive the appropriate treatment. I would like you to keep track of your weight, medication, breathing, and energy level. That way, we will know how you are responding to treatment. In addition, your action plan will tell you when you need to call the office.

Faculty   (*to trainee*) What are you experiencing?

Trainee   Too much information. I would like you to slow down so I can absorb it all.

Faculty   Nice awareness. One way of slowing down and tracking with patients is to use the elicit-provide-elicit format when giving information [1]. Would you like me to review it?

Trainee   Yes, I would.

(continued)

Faculty	The clinician begins the discussion by eliciting the patient's understanding of the condition, "Tell me what you already know or have heard about congestive heart failure." Another way to say it would be, "What do you think would be most important for you to learn about congestive heart failure today?" The clinician provides a chunk of information and then elicits a reaction and understanding. "What are you thinking as you hear all this information?" It is okay if you do not cover everything in one session.
Trainee	I think I have it.
Faculty	Are you ready to go again?
Trainee	Yes

Replay

Trainee	Mr. Smith, I would like to discuss your diagnosis and develop a treatment plan with you today. Is that okay with you?
Patient	Sure.
Trainee	I'm glad your son is here to support you. (*to son*) Let me introduce myself. I'm Dr. Green.
Son	I'm Joe Smith.
Trainee	(*turning to father*) Mr. Smith, tell me what you understand by the term "congestive heart failure."
Patient	I know my heart is not working right—that it is failing.
Trainee	What do you feel when you say your heart is failing?
Patient	Sad.
Trainee	Of course—it is a big loss. Actually, failing is not a good word to describe what is happening [2]. Your heart has not failed or stopped beating. It is pumping blood to your organs, just less strongly. Fatigue and getting short of breath walking around are consequences of this ineffective pumping.
Patient	I'm glad to hear "failing" is not a good description. What can I do about it?
Trainee	We will talk about that in a minute. Let's talk a bit more about the pumping. Just to make sure I have been clear, will you tell me back what I have said so far?
Patient	You said my heart is not pumping well, but it is not completely failing.

(continued)

Trainee	Right. And the shortness of breath when you walk is due to the heart having a difficult time keeping up with the increased oxygen demands of exercise. Your heart is pumping blood with oxygen to your muscles, just not as fast as you are using it.
Patient	I understand.
Trainee	(*to son*) Mr. Smith, do you have any questions?
Son	I'm wondering what caused the heart failure in the first place. My dad has always been so active and healthy.
Trainee	Your dad has cardiomyopathy. We don't know what caused the cardiomyopathy, even after all the testing we have done. It is possible he had a viral infection in the past, and compensated well until his recent symptoms occurred.
Son	It sounds like there is nothing that can be done about it.
Trainee	It is true that the virus that likely caused the cardiomyopathy sometime in the past cannot be treated. However, CHF is treatable. There are a number of ways to help your dad maintain a good quality of life. Let's talk about treatment and develop a plan, Mr. Smith. I will write the plan down so we are all on the same page about how you can stay as healthy as possible.
Patient	That sounds like a good idea.
Son	I live nearby and will be able to help my dad.

Feedback

Faculty	Okay. Let's stop. (*to trainee*) Tell me what you liked about how you interviewed.
Trainee	I think I put into operation the E-P-E format you suggested I use. I asked the patient how he was feeling about the information I was giving him. I gave the information in smaller chunks, and made sure they were with me. I thought we were more of a team.
Faculty	I fully agree. Nice job.

Obstacles to Teaching Concluding Phase

1. Interviewer discounts the amount of time it takes to do a good closing.
2. Interviewer simply tells the patient information, instead of making it a give-and-take format.

Strategies

1. Educate trainees about the importance of separating this phase from the rest of the interview and devoting enough time to do it well. Model good closings to trainees when supervising them.
2. Teach the elicit-provide-elicit structure to trainees.

Concluding Phase[1]

The closing phase of the interview in many primary care settings is routinely short-changed. A clinician can easily spend excessive time on the data gathering stage of an interview and then hurry through the closing phase so that he or she can move to the next patient. Sometimes, a clinician simply discounts the importance of the closing. That is a mistake. The success of the concluding phase largely determines the success of implementing an effective treatment plan [4]. **The importance of this phase should not be undermined by giving quick or premature responses to patients during earlier stages in the interview—when they ask a question or express a self-diagnosis that is leading them to worry.** Their question or worry can be acknowledged by the advisement that you will fully discuss the diagnosis and treatment options after your evaluation. A clinician might respond: *I see you are worried that this might be a clot in her lungs or pneumonia. Lots of conditions can cause these symptoms, most of them not serious. I will talk to you about this as soon as I have all the information I need.* Sometimes, patients are worried about the same diagnosis as we are (e.g., pneumonia). We still can ask them to hold the worry until we get a bit more information. Later we can praise them for their diagnostic acumen and clarify by adding our own ideas.

An effective closing requires the following: time; a thorough knowledge of the diagnosis in question; the ability to explain the condition and treatment in clear, straightforward language; the ability to uncover fears and misperceptions, so they can be discussed and potentially resolved; and the willingness to negotiate. Michael Rothenberg listed five basic questions that must be answered to accomplish the goals of this part of the interview. Sometimes patients and families are too frightened to ask the five basic questions without help from the clinician. These questions provide the framework for the closing:

What do I have?
How did I get it?
Why did I get it?
What is going to be done about it?
What will my course be? [5]

---

[1] Adapted from Binder [3] with permission.

The answers to these questions leads to a shared understanding of the patient's condition. The shared understanding allows for a real partnership in implementing a treatment plan. The patient and family assimilate accurate information only after any distortions they hold regarding the illness are resolved. This makes the closing part of the interview a give-and-take process; the family's understanding is checked each step of the way. In fact, an important first step is to ask the patient or family for their understanding of the condition: *Tell me what you already know or have heard.* This stage might be straightforward for a patient with an ear or sinus infection, but the process remains a give-and-take discussion.

Let us take a look at the process for a family bringing in a child for follow-up after a febrile seizure.

This is a follow up visit for 12-month-old Emily, who was seen two days ago in the ER after a brief febrile seizure. Her development and neurological exam are normal. Parents report no family history of seizures. As the physician sits down to answer the five basic questions for Emily's mother, she notices that Mrs. Phillips' face is drawn and she appears stressed.

Clinician	It sounds like you have had a real stressful week. Tell me what you understand about Emily's condition.
Mother	The emergency room doctor diagnosed a febrile seizure. She seemed well when I put her down for a nap. She became stiff all over. Her color turned blue. It seemed to come out of nowhere.
Comment	*Anything that seems to come out of nowhere is going to be mysterious and upsetting. No wonder Mrs. Phillips is stressed.*
Clinician	It sounds frightening.
Mother	Yes.
Clinician	What worried you the most?
Mother	Her breathing. She was making gurgling noises.
Clinician	Tell me about that.
Mother	I didn't see her breathing. I didn't know what to do.
Clinician	Some parents fear that their child is dying when they witness their child turning blue and having a seizure. Is that true for you? (*third-person technique*)
Mother	I really thought she was dying.
Clinician	And what do you think about that now?
Mother	I stay awake at night thinking of the possibility that Emily might have a seizure and die.
Clinician	No wonder you feel stressed. Let's talk about febrile seizures. Just as people in society communicate with one another, the cells in the brain are connected to other cells in the brain. Cells send messages to one another, using minute amounts of electricity.

(continued)

	This is usually an orderly process. But, problems in sending these messages can occur—just as they do in society. One factor that can make cells misfire in young children is fever [6]. Emily's fever triggered the seizure.
Mother	Why did Emily develop a fever in the first place?
Clinician	We will come back to that as soon as we finish discussing her seizure. Is that okay?
Mother	Yes.
Clinician	Earlier you said you were fearful of Emily having a seizure and dying.
Mother	Yes.
Clinician	During Emily's seizure, her brain cells misfired. This caused her muscles to stiffen, including the muscles controlling her breathing. She was breathing and getting oxygen. She was not dying. Her lips turned blue because the oxygen was going to more important organs than her skin—specifically her brain and heart.
Mother	I didn't realize that.
Trainee	In a recent study of over 300 children who had a seizure and no brain conditions like a stroke, no child died during the five years of the study [7]. I feel confident in saying Emily's risk of dying is no different than a child without a history of febrile seizure. But, I know it can be terrifying to witness a seizure.
Mother	It sure is.
Comment	*Emily's mother appears calmer once her fear has been addressed. The clinician will check her understanding before moving onto the next topic. Patients' recall and comprehension has been estimated to be as low as 50 percent [8]. This is especially likely for patients with low health literacy. Clinicians can reduce this ineffective communication by asking the patient to restate what they heard the clinician say [8].*

Restatement—The patient says back what he has heard the clinician say as a way to check on understanding.

Clinician	To make sure I have explained myself clearly, will you tell me what you heard me say about a benign seizure due to fever? **(restatement)**
Mother	Well, a seizure occurs when the brain cells send too much electricity to other brain cells. This causes the muscles to stiffen.

(continued)

Clinician	Right. And, what about the cause?
Comment	*It is rare for a physician to close the loop—correct any misperceptions so that the patient and doctor have a shared understanding. This may be due to a fear of taking too much time, even though studies show visits are no longer when patient understanding is checked* [8].
Mother	Fever can do it, especially in young children.
Clinician	Okay. What about your scare about what can happen during a benign febrile seizure like Emily experienced? Do you believe you need to stay awake and watch her sleep?
Mother	Not so much. But, I'm still a little worried.
Clinician	Tell me more.
Mother	I believe what you are saying. It is going to take me time to get used to it.
Clinician	Of course.
Comment	*Education is not a one-time event. Families with a chronic condition need re-education throughout the course of the illness.*
Clinician	Let's go over several practical issues. She needs to be watched when she bathes or goes swimming because of the risk of drowning.
Mother	I understand.
Clinician	If she would have another seizure, place her on her side and do not put anything in her mouth. "She will not swallow her tongue" [6]. Most febrile seizures stop within a couple of minutes. If it lasts longer than 5 minutes or recurs, you will need to call an ambulance.
Mother	Okay.
Clinician	Do you have other concerns about Emily's seizure? Some parents have concerns about possible brain damage or even mental retardation [9]. *(third person technique)*
Mother	No, I know she is a smart girl.
Clinician	Earlier you asked about the cause of Emily's fever. *(referred gate)*
Mother	Why did she have a fever?
Clinician	She had a viral infection in her throat causing the fever. The physician in the emergency room examined Emily to make sure her fever was not due to an infection of the brain or its covering.
Mother	Okay. What can I do now about preventing another seizure?
Clinician	We can prevent most febrile seizures if we prescribe a daily medication. I don't recommend that for several reasons. We estimate

(continued)

that Emily has a 70 percent chance she will not experience another febrile seizure [6]. Another febrile seizure would not damage her brain, cause intellectual disability or death as we have already discussed. Medications have the risk of significant side effects, including behavioral problems like being hyperactive. I would not recommend medicine.

Mother	I understand. I didn't want to put Emily on medication.
Clinician	Do you have any more questions?
Mother	Will she have epilepsy when she grows up?
Clinician	Her chance of developing epilepsy is about the same as the chance of children who have never experienced a febrile seizure; there is a 97 % chance that she will not develop epilepsy. The medications we just discussed don't decrease that risk [6]. Before we finish I would like to make a recommendation.
Mother	Please tell me.
Clinician	Set clear limits on her behavior like you would for any child. A temper tantrum because she hears "no" does not cause seizures. Here is a pamphlet on febrile seizures to take home and read. Please call me if you have any questions.
Comment	*An effective closing takes time so that the five basic questions can be asked and answered. When the clinician allots adequate time to each phase of the interview, he or she can smoothly accomplish the goals for the overall encounter.*

Key Points

1. The concluding phase of the interview is often allocated insufficient time.
2. The success of developing a collaborative treatment plan is dependent on this phase.
3. Patient's misconceptions about diagnosis, time course, prognosis, and treatment need to be elicited and discussed.
4. A give-and-take format works best.
5. Restatement enhances partnership by clarifying the patient's understanding.

References

1. Rollnick S, Miller WR, Butler CC. Motivational interviewing in health care: helping patients change behavior. New York, NY: The Guilford Press; 2008.
2. Colucci WS. Heart failure. In: Basow DS, editor. Up to date. Waltham, MA: UpToDate; 2010.
3. Binder J. Pediatric Interviewing: a practical relationship-based approach. New York, NY: Humana Press; 2010.

4. Shea SC. Psychiatric interviewing: the art of understanding: a practical guide for psychiatrists, psychologists, counselors, social workers, nurses, and other mental health professionals. 2nd ed. Philadelphia, PA: W.B. Saunders; 1998.

5. Rothenberg MB. The unholy trinity: activity, authority, and magic. Clin Pediatr. 1974;13:870–3.

6. Freeman JM, Vining EPG, Pillas DJ. Seizures and epilepsy in childhood: a guide for parents. 3rd ed. Baltimore, MD: The Johns Hopkins University Press; 2002.

7. Callenbach MC, Westendorp GJ, Geerts AT, Arts WF, Peeters EA, van Donselaar CA, et al. Mortality risk in children with epilepsy: the Dutch study of epilepsy in childhood. Pediatrics. 2001;107:1259–63.

8. Schillinger D, Piette J, Grumbach K, Wang F, Wilson C, Daher C, et al. Closing the loop: physician communication with diabetic patients who have low health literacy. Arch Intern Med. 2003;163:83–90.

9. Mittan RJ Seizures and epilepsy education program parents' manual: how to raise a child with epilepsy, part 1: coping with fear. EP Mag; 2005 October: 60–66 http://www.eparent.com

Chapter 11
Across the Life Span

James Binder and Michael Binder

Role Play

Prerequisite skills for doing more advanced child, adolescent, and geriatric role plays include *self-awareness, open-ended inquiries*, obtaining *theory of illness*, *eliciting feelings and responding to feelings*, and *identifying strengths/affirmations* (see Introduction and Chaps. 1–8).

Role Play #1: The patient is attending a routine office visit with her mother. She is generally healthy. Typical of many teenagers, she is sporting a nose ring and casual attire. She appears disinterested in the conversation.

Objectives

1. Make an appropriate contract with a 15-year-old girl who is **shut down** at a routine well visit.
2. Maintain a nonjudgmental, friendly approach.

Trainee	I would like to take a minute to get to know you each personally before starting with medical topics. Sarah, would you start by telling me about yourself.
Patient	What do you mean?
Trainee	I would like to know what is important in your life—friends, family, school interests.

(continued)

J. Binder (✉) • M. Binder
Marshall University, School of Medicine, Huntington, WV, USA
e-mail: jbinder2@suddenlink.net

Patient	Not much to say. I'm just a normal teenager.
Mother	That is what she is like at home.
Trainee	Mrs. Payne. Tell me a little about yourself personally.
Mother	I'm a single mother. I have worked hard to give the girls a good home. I work as receptionist in a doctor's office. I get home every night to cook dinner and have family time. Sarah argues with me all the time lately.
Trainee	So you have worked hard to make a good home and now you are having difficulty with Sarah. (*turns to patient*) Sarah is this something you would like to discuss today.
Patient	I don't care.
Trainee	Tell me how you see the situation.
Patient	I don't know.
Trainee	Would you like it to be different?
Patient	I don't care.
Trainee	Well, I will start off hearing from your mother. Sarah, you don't have to talk, but if you want, you can join in.
Mother	I do the best that I can. I am tired when I get home. I ask for simple consideration. Instead, the kitchen is a mess and you, Sarah, are upstairs talking to your friends. What is so great about talking to your friends, anyway? Why don't you talk to me?
Trainee	So you want to reach her and you don't know how.
Mother	Yes. There is not much else I can do.
Patient	You could try talking to me nicely instead of yelling at me.
Mother	I do talk to you nicely.
Patient	What about yesterday, when you got home from work?
Trainee	Let me jump in here for a second. It sounds to me like you both want to connect to each other in a better way. Are you interested in setting that as an initial goal?
Mother	Yes.
Trainee	How about you Sarah.
Patient	Okay.

Feedback

Faculty	Let's stop. Affirmations. (*to trainee*) Why don't you start off with what you thought you did well?
Trainee	I didn't get frustrated and eventually the patient said something. I also thought my rapport with the mother was good.

(continued)

Trainee #2	You kept your cool. Great job.
Patient	I didn't feel you were annoyed with me at all.
Faculty	You didn't take sides. You stayed calm and even. And, you did a beautiful job making a contract and letting the patient decide if and when she wanted to talk. She actually started to open up, and gave her side of the situation.
Trainee	Thanks.
Faculty	Anybody have options?
Group	(*no response*)
Faculty	I don't have any options either.

Role Play #2: An 87 year-old female and her daughter at a routine check-up visit.

Objectives

1. Make an appropriate contract with the patient.
2. Maintain a nonjudgmental, friendly approach, while gathering information to make a functional assessment of patient.

Trainee	Welcome Ms. Goebel. I see you scheduled a comprehensive physical exam. What is most important for us to discuss today?
Patient	I'd like to talk about my diabetes and my blood pressure. I'd also like for you to check my wrist. I tripped at my apartment last week.
Trainee	Is there anything else you'd like to discuss?
Patient	No, that's about it.
Trainee	Before we talk about your medical issues, I would like to get to know you personally. Tell me a little bit about yourself.
Patient	Well, I'm 87, and I'm an independent woman. I've been widowed for over 30 years.
Trainee	Tell me more about yourself.
Patient	I like to go to church on Sundays and eat brunch with some of the people from church after the service each week. I used to read quite a bit, but I don't do as much of that lately because my vision has gotten bad.
Trainee	It sounds like you make it a priority to go to church and to be involved with other people from your church. We know that social

(continued)

	involvement is important to remaining healthy as we age. You mentioned that you fell last week. Tell me more about that.
Patient	It was not that big of a deal. I tripped on the edge of the carpet and jammed my wrist when I hit the floor. It hurt badly for a few days but it's starting to feel better.
Trainee	I'm glad to hear that it's feeling better. How have things been going as far as your diabetes and hypertension are concerned?

Feedback

Faculty	Stop. Let's start with affirmations. (*turns to trainee*) Talk about what you thought you did well.
Trainee	I thought I developed good rapport with the patient. I also thought that I laid the groundwork from the start of our interview about what we were going to address in this clinic visit.
Faculty	I agree. I was also impressed with how you uncovered what is important in her life.
Trainee	Thank you. What can I do better?
Faculty	One option is to ask how her fall has impacted her life. She seemed to minimize it, but that may be because she is embarrassed about it. Let's try that again from the time she talks about her fall.

Replay

Patient	It was not that big of a deal. I tripped on the edge of the carpet and jammed my wrist when I hit the floor. It hurt badly for a few days, but it's starting to feel better.
Trainee	Is that the first time you've fallen?
Patient	No, I've actually fallen several times over the past 6 months or so. I'm spending more time indoors.
Trainee	You are spending more time indoors because of your falls?
Patient	Yes. My daughter helps me out by picking up groceries each week. I used to do all my own grocery shopping but I don't go out as much now because I'm fearful of falling.
Trainee	What are you most scared about?

(continued)

Patient	I'm scared that I'll really hurt myself if I fall again. Next time it might not be just a sprain or a bruise.
Patient	I'm scared that I'll really hurt myself if I fall again. Next time it might not be just a sprain or a bruise.
Trainee	Are there other ways that you've dealt with your falls?
Patient	No, I'm not sure what else I can do besides taking it easy.
Trainee	Maybe we could problem solve this with the help of your daughter. Would that be okay with you?
Patient	Sure. She is in the waiting room.
Trainee	Great. I'll invite her in for the visit.

Feedback

Faculty	Let's stop there. (*turns to trainee*) How do you think that went?
Trainee	I thought that line of questioning led to a better understanding of how these falls have impacted her independence. At first, she seemed to dismiss them. By digging a little bit deeper, I found out that wasn't the case at all.
Faculty	Remember, assessment of functioning is a key step to being able to help the geriatric patient.

Obstacles to Teaching Interviewing Across the Life Span

1. Interviewer lacks knowledge of key communication and developmental capacities of childhood, adolescence, and old age.
2. Interviewer discounts the importance of direct communication with child or geriatric patients.
3. Interviewer has no experience in the pragmatics of communicating with young children.
4. Interviewer assumes adolescents can be engaged in the same manner as adults.
5. Interviewer discounts the importance of independence and self-worth to the elderly.
6. Interviewer has a negative stereotype of the elderly.
7. Interviewer's family-of-origin issues interfere with healthy communication (e.g., that elderly man acts just like my grandpa).

Strategies

1. Integrate the teaching of development into the interviewing curriculum.
2. Educate trainers regarding the research showing health benefits of direct communication with children and geriatric patients.

3. Give trainers specific statements or questions to use with small children. Have them observe at a good preschool.
4. Encourage trainees to stretch themselves—risking vulnerability can lead to growth.
5. Teach trainers a three-phase method for structuring interviews with adolescents. Explain the rationale.
6. Expose trainees to clinicians who have positive attitudes towards the elderly.
7. Address self-awareness issues. Help trainees with family-of-origin issues in small groups.

Across the Life Cycle

The capacity to create solid engagement with individuals across the entire life cycle is an essential skill for primary care clinicians. Partnership is a prerequisite to helping people make good healthcare decisions at all ages. Direct communication with the patient and with each family member present is essential. The core interviewing skills required to build a good relationships do not change with age: being emotionally present to the patient; maintaining nonjudgmental respect; inviting the patient to tell his or her story; listening carefully; eliciting and acknowledging the emotional experience of the patient; identifying strengths; and affirming the patient. However, interviewing techniques must be adapted to the communication and developmental capacities of individuals at both ends of the age spectrum—for young children and for the elderly. Several unique aspects of talking with young children, adolescents, and geriatric patients will be considered in this chapter.

Preschool Children

The main developmental task of the preschool child is to learn about the world by initiating social interactions and activities. The preschooler takes great pleasure in his or her capacity to initiate patterns of interaction that are copied from adults and replayed over and over again in play. Magical thinking and egocentrism are at the center of the preschool child's perception of reality [1]. Magical thinking helps a preschooler cope with the demands of managing life as a 3–6-year-old child. It also places the child at risk for fears of imagined danger (e.g., *I was put into the hospital because I was mean to my sister*).

Although preschoolers don't possess the capacity for scientific thinking, they are capable of learning about their illnesses in a concrete way and participating in good self-care [2]. Preschoolers learn through seeing and doing—not through words alone [3]. Drawing a picture and having a conversation about it give the preschooler a visual image of his or her illness. A parent of a child with cystic fibrosis might draw a picture of the lungs and paint dots in the bottom of the lungs to represent bugs (bacteria). Different colored dots are painted to represent medication dramatically killing the bugs [3]. Understanding helps the child begin to develop a sense of control and mastery.

Play is the gateway to connection with the preschooler [4]. A clinician can position him or herself at eye level to avoid the appearance of being a large, scary adult looking down at the child. An animated, friendly approach works better than a strict question and answer format. Comments about specific people or events in the preschooler's life, such as a birthday party or a favorite superhero, open up the conversation [4, 5]. Reflective statements (*You have a big dog!*) and affirmations (*You have strong muscles!*) help maintain a lively conversation.

If a child appears anxious, a slower pace and quieter tone might better mirror his or her demeanor. The third-person technique can be adapted to help an anxious child of this age. For example, *I know a little girl who gets scared when she goes to the doctor. Does that happen with you?*

School-Aged Children

A supportive family provides the secure base from which the school-aged child manages the demands of the outside world and develops a sense of competence. Acquiring competence in academics, peer relationships, and group activities is the key developmental task of the school-aged child. It is often useful to initiate a conversation by expressing interest in one of these areas, such as with: *What a colorful jersey. Do you play soccer?* Once the child is engaged, discovering the important people and things in the child's life allows the clinician to learn about this unique individual and build their relationship [6].

Rider suggests the following questions [5]:

What do you like to do with mom? With dad?
Tell me about your friends.
What do you like to do with your friends?
Who do you talk to if you have worries?

A mix of open-ended and closed-ended questions feels comfortable to most school-aged children visiting the doctor. Identifying strengths—asking about the things they do well—contributes to a supportive atmosphere. A child will be a more willing to partner with the clinician on health issues in the future if he or she has first developed a trusting relationship with the clinician [6]. School-aged children are typically capable of providing sequential details of their illness and participating with the clinician in treatment [1]. For example, a child with encopresis might be encouraged: *Take your medicine... It will help make the muscles in your intestines become stronger!*

Adolescence

Adolescent behavior is best understood within the context of creating a deeper sense of identity as children move from dependency to independency [7]. Developing an autonomous self is the main developmental task of adolescence. The first step in achieving autonomy is questioning adult norms. Distrust of adult traditions and values can make communication with adolescents challenging. A thoughtful approach, one that is responsive to the developmental context, is needed. The following three-step approach, similar to the structure suggested for sensitive topics is one such method.

1. Self-check for any thoughts that might interfere with a strong engagement with adolescents or their parents.
2. Set the stage.
3. Move from less sensitive to more sensitive topics, utilizing normalization techniques to decrease anxiety.

Interfering Cognitions

Clinicians can best help adolescents and their families when they avoid alliances with either the adolescent or his or her parents. A compassionate and accepting attitude with both adolescents and parents is needed. Family-of-origin issues can trigger reactions in clinicians that threaten this balanced approach.

> A young clinician is taking care of a 15-year-old adolescent who is experimenting with the use of alcohol. His parents are anxious and controlling. The clinician grew up with authoritarian parents and he attempted to please them. He finds himself having a very difficult time joining with the 15-year-old adolescent. He thinks: *What a rotten kid!* He remains unaware of his prejudices until he seeks a consultation in the role play group about his difficulty joining with teenagers.

Consultation with colleagues can help clinicians broaden their perspective and approach families more effectively [8].

We know (from studies asking adolescents directly) what is required to build a trusting relationship with most adolescents. The interviewer must be friendly, unpretentious, and not rushed [9]. The adolescent needs time to assess whether it will be safe to talk to this adult about important matters. A nonjudgmental stance is essential. This requires the clinician to resolve any prejudicial beliefs, like the one above.

Set the Stage

The second step of the interview has two elements:

1. Make a contract for the visit.
2. Begin the conversation with nonsensitive subject material before moving to personal questions.

The clinician must ask personal questions of the adolescent since the greatest risks to his or her health involve personal topics: sex, alcohol, drugs, depression, suicide, and violence [10]. The adolescent is not likely to have planned on discussing these topics when visiting the physician. However, good medical care demands that they be addressed. Adolescents will more likely answer these questions openly if they understand why the clinician is asking the questions [11]. A clear contract with an adolescent includes the rationale for asking personal questions and a discussion of privacy so that an adolescent knows it is safe to be open with the clinician. A sample contract to be discussed with an adolescent and the adolescent's parents might go like this [12]:

Clinician	Tom, now that you are older and can take more responsibility for keeping yourself healthy, it is important that we talk about how the visits will go. I would like to talk with you alone during part of the visit. The reason for that is to give you privacy when I ask you questions, some of which may be personal. As your doctor I am interested in seeing you when you have a sore throat. I am also interested in helping you deal with all the things that can affect a teenager's health—things like sex, stress, depression, alcohol, and drugs. I know these topics are usually private and can be hard to talk about. You have a free choice to talk with me or not. I will not tell your parents or anyone else about what you tell me. The only exception would be a situation in which your life or someone else's life was in immediate danger. For example, if you were planning to kill yourself; in such a case, I would talk to your parents to find ways to help you. My goal is to help you be healthy. I can best do that if you are open and honest with me. Is this agreeable with you, Tom?
Patient	Yes
Clinician	Mr. and Mrs. Green, is that arrangement okay with you?
Parents	Yes, we want him to have someone we trust to whom he can talk.
Clinician	Great.

Once a contract has been finalized, the clinician transitions to the biomedical part of the history. Starting in a nonsensitive area lessens any anxiety the adolescent might be experiencing before more personal questions are asked.

Third Phase

Transition to the third phase of the interview follows directly upon completion of the biomedical part of the history. Initial inquiries into school, friends, and activities are followed by assessment of sensitive and high-risk behaviors. Sequencing questioning in that order reduces discomfort [12]. Acknowledging the adolescent's strengths (*It sounds like you make friends easily*) throughout the conversation solidifies engagement and enhances a sense that it is safe to talk.

Shut Down Adolescent

Some adolescents will not open up despite skilled use of the above strategies. The adolescent will be slow to respond, answer with unintelligible monosyllables, look disinterested, and even repeat the phrase "I don't know" to simple questions. The shutdown interview can trigger frustration and anxiety in almost any clinician. Surprisingly, the interview is not necessarily doomed. The clinician has reasonably effective options. If the clinician views the shutdown interview as a challenge and an opportunity rather than a personal rejection, he or she is free to respond in any number of ways:

1. The clinician can do a quick self-assessment. Is he or she conveying frustration or annoyance? If so, this can be resolved by recognizing that the adolescent is simply being an adolescent. **It is not personal**.
2. Using his or her other intuition, the clinician might imagine what this adolescent is feeling emotionally and attempt to connect with him or her.

   Is this adolescent simply shy and just need time to warm up?
   Is he or she depressed?
   Is he or she feeling shame about a medical condition?
   Is this adolescent a rebellious teenager?

   The clinician intuits what the adolescent is feeling by paying attention to nonverbal communication. An adolescent, who pushes back in his chair and turns his head down and away, might be depressed. A shy teenager might speak softly, and a rebellious or angry teenager might snap back with short, clipped responses. Since it is only an intuition, the clinician will need corroborating evidence. The third-person technique allows the clinician to make an inquiry in a nonconfrontational way [13].

   Adolescent appearing quiet and sad:

Clinician	Some kids find themselves getting down in the dumps—feeling blue and depressed. They feel bad, but find it hard to talk to an adult about it. Is that true for you?

Adolescent appears rebellious:

Clinician	Lots of adolescents don't like to go to the doctor. They think to themselves, "You can make me go, but you can't make me talk." Is that true for you?

Adolescent appears shy:

Clinician	Many people your age find themselves feeling nervous, a little bit worried, when they have to go to the doctor. Do you feel that way?
Comment	*Since the anxious or shy teen needs time to warm up, it is often best to begin with questions that require only brief responses.*

A positive response to any of the above inquiries is tracked and expanded, until a stronger engagement is achieved.

3. The clinician can offer the adolescent a new contract [14].

Patient	(*silence*)
Clinician	It is okay if you don't talk. I'll talk to your parents and you join in if you change your mind.

This contract simply makes overt what the adolescent is already doing. If the adolescent is feeling rebellious, he or she has nothing to rebel against. Often, after the adolescent hears what his parents have to say, he or she will want to join in the conversation. It can be a very effective maneuver. It is my personal favorite.

4. Finally, the clinician can talk with the adolescent about any topic the adolescent seems interested in discussing [15]. It is important that the clinician be genuinely interested and not rush him or her. This phase of the interview is not a task to be accomplished in order to get to the real agenda. Joining is part of the agenda and it takes time with a shutdown adolescent.

Geriatric Medicine

Engaging, partnering, and guiding the interview to understand and help solve problems are the basic principles of interviewing older adults, just as for younger patients. Barriers to accomplishing these goals with geriatric patients include:

- A focus on multiple diseases instead of the **functional** impact on the patient.
- Disregarding the importance of family input.
- Interfering beliefs of the interviewer.
- Sensory and communication deficits.

Consider the case of an 88 year-old man with diabetes who comes in for a routine office visit to the resident clinic:

John has been a widower for 22 years. Until recently he shopped and prepared his own meals. He spent his time gardening, reading and watching television. His son and daughter-in-law live in town and talk to him daily on the phone. He is a friendly person.

Clinician	Welcome, how have things been going with you since your last office visit?
Patient	Everything has been going well.
Clinician	How about your blood sugars, what have they been like?
Patient	They've been normal.
Clinician	That is good to hear. Did you take you medicines already today?
Patient	Yes, I always take my medications.

Comprehensive Assessment

This friendly patient answered all the questions appropriately, but he did not provide details. The busy resident mistook the friendliness as evidence that the patient was cognitively intact. He regarded him as an easy patient, who would allow him to quickly move to the next patient. The patient's hemoglobin A1c had increased from 7 to 9 % in the last 6 months. The resident simply increased the dose of insulin. He did not uncover that this man was in the early stage of dementia and was not taking his insulin as prescribed. His treatment placed his patient in danger. This mistake could have been avoided by an inquiry into cognitive and functional problems that affect the elderly. Formal comprehensive geriatric assessments by multidisciplinary teams have been proven to lower mortality rates, as well as to enhance the cognitive and functional status of adults with complex medical problems [16].

Most elderly patients with dementia are not recognized by their primary care physicians [17]. Depression and substance abuse are also common and easy to overlook. Priorities shift when patients age. The long-term consequences of diseases like diabetes and hypertension are no longer high priorities. The patient's functional status takes on increased importance. The clinician must ask him or herself how the medical condition impacts the ability of the patient to perform activities of daily living independently and enjoy life. Part of the standard assessment of geriatric patients should include psychosocial screening for conditions such as dementia, substance abuse, insomnia, and depression. Other medical issues that commonly impair functioning in geriatric patients include poor nutrition, treatment with multiple medications, memory loss, urinary incontinence, and falls, as in the patient above. Prioritizing and focusing on the problems that interfere with functioning are key to positive outcomes with geriatric patients.

Family Involvement

For the patient in the vignette above, it was difficult to achieve a clear picture of his functional status without collateral information. Obtaining input from the family is vital. Family members can be an invaluable resource. When family members accompany patients to clinic visits, we suggest partnering with them. When they are not at the visit, but might be supportive, we encourage inviting them to the next exam. It is important to avoid forming coalitions during family interviews. (See Chap. 13 for further development of coalitions.)

Other Barriers

Sensory issues are common among the geriatric population. Hearing problems affect over half of people over age 65 [18]. Hearing loss can lead to social isolation and depression. The clinician has a number of techniques available to improve communication with the hearing impaired: make good eye contact; speak at a moderate rate without background distractions; pause at the end of sentences and do not drop words; and inform patients when changing the subject [19].

Blocks to communication also originate in the interviewer. The clinician may hold a belief that interferes with effective care. In the above case, the clinician thought a friendly demeanor ruled out dementia. There are any number of beliefs that underlie ageism, such as: *Older people naturally lose their independence*; *The elderly do not have much to offer, other than a list of medical problems; Successfully managing a medical problem in very old patient does not make much of a difference in the patient's life*. The astute clinician stays aware and resolves such blocks to a solid engagement with his or her patient.

Key Points

1. Play is the gateway to connection with the preschooler.
2. School-aged children are involved in family, school, and group activities. A conversation can be initiated by expressing an interest in one of those areas.
3. The clinician builds a relationship with the school-aged child by discovering the important people and things in the child's life.
4. Providing health care to adolescents involves the discussion of sensitive issues. Establishing a clear contract about what is going to be discussed during the visit, including confidentiality, is essential.
5. The care of geriatric patients requires specific knowledge, extra time, and a clear strategy to address common barriers to data collection, such as hearing problems or slow, rambling communication (see Chap. 9 for a discussion of rambling).
6. The elderly usually have multiple medical problems. It is important to perform a systematic assessment with emphasis on functional impairment.

References

1. Sattler JM. Clinical and forensic interviewing of children and families. Guidelines for the mental health, education, pediatric, and child maltreatment fields. San Diego, CA: Jerome M. Sattler; 1998.
2. Holzheimer L, Mohay H, Masters IB. Educating young children about asthma: comparing the effectiveness of a developmentally appropriate asthma education videotape and picture book. Child Care Health Dev. 1998;24:85–99.
3. Cline FW, Greene LC. Parenting children with health issues. Golden, CO: Love and Logic Press; 2007.
4. Rider EA. The examination. Arch Pediatr Adolesc Med. 2005;159:414.
5. Rider EA. Communication and relationships with children and parents. In: Novack DH, Clark WD, Daetwyler C, Saizow DB, editors. doc.com – an interactive learning resource for health-care communication [Internet]. Philadelphia, PA: American Academy on Communication in healthcare/Drexel University College of Medicine. Accessed on 17 Mar 2012. http://www.AACHonline.org.
6. The Bayer-Fetzer Conference on Physician-Patient Communication in Medical Education. Essential elements of communication in medical encounters: the Kalamazoo Consensus Statement. Acad Med. 2001;76:390–3.
7. Cline F, Fay J. Parenting teens with love and logic: preparing adolescents for responsible adulthood. 2nd ed. Colorado Springs, CO: Nav Press; 2006.
8. McDaniel SH, Bank J, Campbell TL, Mancini J, Shore B. Using a group as a consultant. In: Wynne L, McDaniel SH, Weber T, editors. Systems consultation: a new perspective for family therapy. New York, NY: The Guilford Press; 1986.
9. Malus M, LaChance PA, Lamy L, Macaulay A, Vanasse M. Priorities in adolescent health care: the teenager's viewpoint. J Fam Pract. 1987;25:159–62.
10. Millstein S, Irwin C, Adler N, Cohn L, Kegeles S, Dolcini M. Health-risk behaviors and health concerns among young adolescents. Pediatrics. 1992;3:422–78.
11. Platt FW, Gordon GH. Field guide to the difficult patient interview. 2nd ed. Philadelphia, PA: Lippincott Williams and Wilkins; 2004.

12. Ginsberg K. The adolescent interview. In: Novack DH, Clark WD, Daetwyler C, Saizow DB, editors. doc.com – an interactive learning resource for healthcare communication [Internet]. Philadelphia, PA: American Academy on Communication in healthcare/Drexel University College of Medicine. Accessed 17 Mar 2012. http://www.AACHonline.org.

13. Kohlberg I, Rothenberg MB. Comprehensive care following multiple life-threatening injuries. Am J Dis Child. 1970;119:449–51.

14. Anderson CM, Stewart S. Mastering resistance: a practical guide to family therapy. New York, NY: The Guilford Press; 1983.

15. Shea SC. Psychiatric interviewing: the art of understanding: a practical guide for psychiatrists, psychologists, counselors, social workers, nurses and other health professionals. 2nd ed. Philadelphia, PA: WB Saunders; 1998.

16. Wells JL, Seabrook JA, Stolee P, Borrie MJ, Knoefel F. State of the art in geriatric rehabilitation. Part II: clinical challenges. Arch Phys Med Rehabil. 2003;84:898–903.

17. Finkel SI. Cognitive screening in the primary care setting: the role of physicians at the first point of entry. Geriatrics. 2003;58:43–4.

18. Mader SL. Hearing impairment in the elderly. J Am Geriatr Soc. 1984;32:542–53.

19. Mader SL, Ford AB. The geriatric interview. In: Lipkin M, Putnam SM, Lazare A, editors. The medical interview: clinical care, education, and research. New York, NY: Springer; 1995.

Part II
Teaching Complex Interviewing Skills

The complex interviewing skills discussed in the remainder of the book assume mastery (and continued practice) of the basic skills taught in Part I. The trainee must now develop the ability to sequence skills. Greater flexibility is required. Constructive feedback and repetition of role play to a level of competence ensure that learning is progressing.

Macrotraining is an educational tool that was specifically developed to teach complex interviewing skills (e.g., suicide assessment, domestic violence assessment, etc.) to psychiatric residents and other professionals [1]. Serial role play, with each new role play incorporating previously learned material, is the key teaching strategy of macrotraining [1]. The repetition reinforces skill acquisition. Serial role play is strongly recommended for the complex skills covered in Part II of this text. For example, imagine that primary care residents have the goal of learning how to assess depression. The following steps would be taught in one long workshop or in weekly hour-long sessions. The steps:

1. Screen for depression
2. Elicit and respond to feelings (a review)
3. Invite patient to tell his story of depression and deepen story
4. Ask about neurovegetative symptoms and signs
5. Ask questions needed to develop a solid differential diagnosis
6. Validity techniques (a review)
7. Assess suicide (a full suicide assessment would be learned in a separate macrotraining)

After each step is learned, the trainee does another role play front to back until a level of competency is reached.

Reference

1. Shea SC, Barney C. Macrotraining: a "how to" primer for using serial role-playing to train complex clinical interviewing tasks such as suicide assessment. Psychiatr Clin N Am. 2007;30:e1–20.

Chapter 12
Family Concepts

This chapter provides a thumbnail sketch of general family concepts, followed by a description of the different ways primary care clinicians can be involved with families. This very brief overview is intended to be an introduction for the primary care trainee who will begin family interviewing role plays. The references at the end of this chapter are a starting point for those interested in reading about the theoretical aspects of family interviewing.

1. Family characteristics.
2. Ways primary care clinicians can be involved with families.

Kadis and McClendon define family "to be a group of people who have a kinship bond and currently share a common experience" [1]. They use the metaphor of a car engine to help the reader visualize each family as a system. Just as the individual parts (cylinders, pistons, etc.) of a car engine spread out end to end on a garage floor do not make an engine, so, too, with the individual members of a family [1]. In any system, such as a family, one part influences and is influenced by other parts. For example, a wife may believe her husband does not spend enough time with their children and anxiously tells him to spend more time with them. Only the husband perceives this as hassling. He responds by pouting and spending less time with the children, which increases his wife's anxiety and reminders. If either of them would change their response, the negative cycle could be broken. If the wife remained warm and playful, the husband would be more likely to become engaged with her and the children; if the husband stopped pouting and became curious about his wife's anxiety, she would probably calm down [2].

Family members influence a patient's health-related behaviors and health outcomes more strongly than other social factors [3]. Patients with schizophrenia, depression, diabetes mellitus, and asthma all do worse in the context of a critical family environment [4–6]. Nurturing environments improve the health of patients—no surprise there! [3] An effective primary care clinician harnesses the power in families to improve the health of his or her patients.

J. Binder, *Primary Care Interviewing: Learning Through Role Play*,
DOI 10.1007/978-1-4614-7224-7_12, © Springer Science+Business Media New York 2013

Research supports the claim that family-oriented interventions change health outcomes. Education, psycho-education (focus on helping families cope with an illness), and family therapy approaches have all been shown to be effective. In one representative study of hypertensive patients, counseling the spouse during a home visit resulted in a significant reduction in blood pressure and a 50 % reduction in mortality [7]. It is no wonder that the National Heart, Lung, and Blood Institute recommends involving an influential family member in treatment of hypertension [8]. A review of the medical family literature leads to one conclusion: optimal health care requires a family orientation [6].

A family-focused clinician considers a family from a number of perspectives: level of functioning, structure, process, movement through time, and cultural background. The following very brief description of these five dimensions provides a framework for conceptualizing "family." The more deeply a clinician understands these five dimensions in a particular family, the more likely he or she will be able to develop a strong engagement with the family, hear their concerns and problems, and help them move in a positive direction.

Level of Functioning

The ability of a family to support its members successfully differentiating and achieving the expected tasks of each stage of the life cycle (school, work, marriage) equates with the level of functioning of a family. Individuals in families functioning at a lower developmental level—as distinct from a lower socioeconomic level— have difficulty expressing their feelings and needs directly. They do not resolve problems well because they also struggle to listen supportively to each other. Commonly, these families present clinically either in uproar or in a withdrawn, agitated state. Family members carry diagnoses such as substance abuse, domestic violence, personality disorder, or a serious medical condition. Histories of emotional trauma or other trauma are frequently present. Family members often resist looking at their own contribution to family turmoil [9].

Not only did these family members grow up with a lack of emotional support, they typically did not understand why people were acting the way they were. They received a lack of clear explanation for people's actions. Futility and helplessness followed. It is important for clinicians to tell these families what they are doing and why they are doing it: *Learning to listen to each other will help you develop better relationships.* Education, coaching, and a warm, empathic approach by the clinician can help families change their attitude about the possibility of change [10]. Highly distressed families are not going to be able to solve problems until they believe that they can solve them (and learn a different *process* for managing their differences) [10]. These families also need [9]:

1. **Consistency and reliability over time**, in order to develop trust in the clinician.
2. **Affirmations** for what they are doing well.

3. **A developmental, process-oriented approach**. For example, if a family member does not know how to listen to other members, it is premature to expect this member to be empathic. It can be easy to overestimate the developmental level of a family member who appears educated or intellectually sophisticated.
4. **Problems broken into manageable segments**. Highly distressed families often respond better to concrete communication, rather than the introspection characteristic of traditional therapy [11].

Higher functioning families typically present with adjustment problems—adjustment to a new illness, or a change in the developmental phase of the family. They are capable of talking out problems and resolving them, sometimes with support from professionals.

Families exist at all points between these two extremes of functioning. A number of assessment tools are available to help the clinician place the family accurately on that spectrum [1, 9].

Structure

Salvador Minuchin referred to the organization underlying family interactions as the structure of the family. He divided the family into subsystems—spousal, parental, and siblings—with boundaries separating the different subsystems, as well as the generations. Boundaries are defined as the unwritten rules that establish the hierarchy of relationships in the family. That is, how, when, and with whom family members relate. The boundaries function clearly (healthy), rigidly (which restricts the ability of family members to ask for needed support), or diffusely (which undermines the ability of family members to operate autonomously and develop a sense of mastery) [12].

A common structural issue in alcoholic families is a reversal of roles [13]. An older child takes on parental responsibilities (e.g., supervising younger children neglected by the parents). This child helps solve a family problem, but at the cost of giving up a large part of his or her childhood. It is a big loss. Another frequent structural variation, especially in families with children acting out behaviorally and emotionally, is a coalition. A parent, having emotional difficulty with his or her spouse, colludes with a child against the spouse [14].

Minuchin emphasized the importance of joining and accommodating to families and then developing behavioral interventions, challenging families to change. Once the family restructured itself, symptoms in the index patient would abate. Minuchin successfully treated multiproblem families, who often had little psychological insight, with this behavioral approach [11].

Family Process

The interpersonal process, as opposed to content, has to do with the way communication is expressed—the nonverbal communication, and the tone of the verbal communication:

- How does the family arrange themselves in the room?
- How are they dressed?
- What are their body postures?
- What are their facial expressions?
- What is the general feeling tone?
- Who talks to whom?
- Who begins to tell the story?
- What are their feelings?
- Are family members close? Distant? [15]

Many clinicians have not been trained to pay attention to process [15]. With practice, they learn to describe interpersonal processes. Interpersonal processes can be analyzed by assessing family members using the following parameters:

Differentiation

Differentiation refers to a family member's growth process: the ability to think his or her own thoughts and feel his or her own emotions. When differentiation is supported by a family, family members learn to take responsibility for their own thoughts and feelings, and take action to get their needs met directly. This allows them more flexibility in solving problems. It also avoids the dysfunctional communication patterns that result from two people behaving as though they were one person [14].

Basic Belief About Okayness

"Okayness" has to do with an individual's belief about his or her own essential nature and is the driving force underlying his or her behavior and life experience [14]. Children who believe they are "okay" act in positive ways; children who believe they are "not okay" exhibit negative behaviors.

Stroking Pattern

In Transactional Analysis terminology, a stroke is "any act implying recognition of another's presence" [16]. The type (positive or negative, conditional, or unconditional) and frequency are noted. A paucity of strokes or an increased ratio of negative strokes might be present in a depressed family. Often parents inadvertently reinforce negative behavior by stroking it. For example, a parent makes a comment every time a child makes a mistake and ignores positive behavior. Vann Joines notes that "Changing the stroking pattern allows the members to reinforce a different kind of behavior. Until the stroking pattern is changed, it is difficult for individuals in the family to change, because they are being reinforced for their typical behaviors" [14].

Family Mood

Many families have a prevailing mood such as depression, anxiety, or frustration, which has been reinforced time and again within the family [14]. If the prevailing mood is frustration, it is likely members respond to an individual's frustration, but not when the member is sad or happy.

Family Through Time

The family is an emotional system that connects members separated geographically. Carter and McGoldrick emphasize that the emotional life of a family includes three or four generations of people. Members of one household react to past, present, and even anticipated future relationships within that family system [17]. Family events, such as trauma, a cutoff, or a childhood death, can have powerful effects on future generations. New members continue to arrive into the family via birth and adoption; members leave only by death [17].

The genogram is a practical tool that allows the clinician to quickly visualize family relationships and patterns—essential information for a family-oriented clinician. The basic information for the genogram can be recorded when the family history is taken at the initial visit. Details can be added at future visits [3].

Each generation of the family moves through predictable stages, as it realigns to support the entry, development, and launching of individual members. A young adult separates from his or her own parents, marries, becomes a parent, raises, and then launches children of his or her own. Each stage in the life cycle is associated with key tasks that must be accomplished in order to move through the stage successfully [17]. Families must change and adapt. It is at these nodal points in the lifestyle that families typically get stuck and present with clinical symptoms.

Parents of a family in the adolescent stage may have difficulty supporting independence and autonomy in their adolescent, while staying emotionally connected. This is particularly challenging for the adolescent with a chronic illness, such as diabetes mellitus or severe asthma [17].

Cultural Humility

Cultural influences on a patient's health beliefs and behaviors are particularly important in the United States at this time. Efforts to improve cultural sensitivity have often focused on teaching the beliefs, attitudes, and values of various ethnic groups. Specific approaches to various groups were recommended; other approaches were to be avoided [18]. For example, maintaining direct eye contact with people from certain Asian countries was to be avoided. Although valuable, this approach proved problematic. Cultures evolved and old patterns changed. More importantly, although many members of a culture might share a characteristic, individuals possess their own unique way of being in this world. Approaching all members of a group as if they are the same leads to stereotyping [18].

Patient-centered care avoids both of the above problems. Patient-centered care focuses on the values, needs, and preferences of the individual. Cultural traditions, preferences, and lifestyles are taken into account. The patient and family share in decision making. Patient-centered care is associated with decreased health disparities because of better communication [18].

Betancourt suggests clinicians learn a framework for providing culturally sensitive care to patients and families that supports effective communication in any culture. One such framework is the ESFT (Explanatory, Social Risk, Fears, Therapeutic Contracting) model. Questions are asked in each of four categories to elicit information needed to address cultural differences [18, 19]. The specifics of the clinical situation will dictate which questions are selected for a given patient.

Explanatory Model of Health and Wellness

- *What do you think caused your problems?*
- *Why do you think it started when it did?*
- *How does it affect you?*
- *What worries you most?*
- *What kind of treatment do you think you should receive?*

Social and Environmental Factors Affecting Adherence

- *How do you get your medications?*
- *Are they difficult to afford?*
- *Do you have time to pick them up?*
- *How quickly do you get them?*
- *Do you have help getting them if you need it?*

Fears and Concerns About Medication and Side Effects

- *Are you concerned with the dosage, color, or size of the pill?*
- *Have you heard anything about this medication?*
- *Are you worried about side effects?*

Treatment Understanding

- *Do you understand how to take the medication? Can you tell me how to take it?*
  [18, p. 58]

Establishing safety and trust, the core of every healthy relationship, can be a challenge when patients have been raised in a different culture. They may have beliefs or experiences that influence them not to trust the clinician [19]. Once the threat to trust is made explicit, it can be discussed and efforts made to solidify trust.

Clinician	I know that we come from different cultures. Sometimes in that situation, a person is not sure how the doctor might ask questions, figure out what to do, or even how the doctor might use the information he gets. Is that true for you?
Patient	In my country, it is different.
Clinician	How is it different?

The curious clinician asks about differences between medical care in their country of origin and the United States, and about the way family or friends view the problem. At the conclusion of the visit, it is important to ask the patient if he or she can think of anything that would make it difficult to follow the treatment plan [19].

Clinical Level of Involvement

Doherty and Baird describe five levels of clinician involvement with families [20]. Clinicians communicate with families in mostly biomedical terms at the first two levels. Medical issues are discussed with families. A biopsychosocial approach is characteristic of levels three, four, and five. Clinicians operating at level three or above elicit the feelings and concerns of family members, normalize families' reactions to illness, express empathy, provide psychoeducation, and are generally solidly supportive of families. Primary care trainees certainly can and should learn how to function competently at level three.

Clinicians operating at level four assess family dynamics and the impact of the illness on the family and then intervene in ways to help the family change the interaction patterns. They help the family utilize its strengths and resources to solve problems. The problems are not complex or long-standing—typically, an adjustment to an illness or a change in the family development cycle. Trainees need a comprehensive family interviewing curriculum, including supervision with real families, to move to level four. In such a program, a trainee might present a family from his clinic to the supervisory person or team.

> Case: a 57-year-old woman has chronic musculoskeletal pain. Her husband offered suggestions at first, but that did not help the situation. He has coped by withdrawing, becoming passive and resentful. The patient, in turn, has had increased pain. The trainee suggests that she bring her husband to the next visit. The supervisor teaches the trainee how to mirror back to the couple their destructive communication cycle. The trainee then learns how to move them through their stuck place to a more effective way of communicating their feelings.

Clinicians working at level five are trained family therapists dealing with deeply rooted and complex family problems. This book focuses on using role plays to teach skills for interviewing families at level three. Once trainees have mastered these skills, they will have the foundation needed to learn advanced family interviewing techniques and strategies.

Forms of a Family Visit[1]

Routine Family Office Visits

A routine office visit is the more common form of visit that clinicians have with families. Family members frequently accompany patients to the doctor visit. Including family members in health care takes only a few extra minutes, except in unusual circumstances. They help in a number of ways: communicate patient concerns, improve data collection, support the patient's understanding of his or her illness, encourage lifestyle changes or adherence to treatment recommendations, as well as express their own concerns about the patient and what the impact of the illness has been on the family [3]. When the clinician understands a family member's feelings and concerns, he or she can address them, so they do not undermine the patient's treatment at home. The family then becomes the clinician's ally in treatment.

The clinician can set up his or her office so that family members feel invited to participate-signs in the office, family members greeted warmly, and the availability of physical space for families to participate [3]. McDaniel et al. [3] recommend including the family routinely in five specific clinical settings.

---

[1]Forms of a Family Visit are adapted from McDaniel et al. [3] with permission.

Routine Obstetrical and Well-Child Care

Clinicians should encourage fathers to be included in obstetrics to discuss the pregnancy and labor; and, invite them at least once for well-child care to assess how the family is adjusting to the transition. A clinician might call and say to the father: *In providing health care to babies, I find it important for me to get to know the father's perspective on how the baby and family are adjusting. Would you be willing to come to the next check-up with the baby and your wife?*

Diagnosis of a Serious Chronic Illness

Adapting to a chronic condition like diabetes mellitus can be incredibly challenging for patients and families. Some families under function, while others over function, overprotect, and develop conflict. The clinician has an opportunity to help families cope with improved communication and closeness.

Noncompliance with Treatment Recommendations

When a family supports a medical treatment, the patient is more likely to follow the treatment plan; conversely, when a family criticizes a treatment plan, the patient is much less likely to stick with treatment. This is true for medication treatments and lifestyle changes, such as smoking cessation. Including family members allows the clinician to solicit family support for his or her treatment recommendations.

Somatization or Unexplained Medical Symptoms

Patients with unexplained physical symptoms often avoid discussion of psycho-social problems. Having other family members present can sometimes help the clinician expand the focus beyond the physical by their willingness to address interpersonal issues.

Health Problems that Have a Significant Interpersonal Component

Relationship problems both contribute to and result from mental conditions. Meeting with family members helps the clinician to understand the problems more fully, leading to better solutions.

Many psychosocial problems require more than one 15-min office visit. Primary care clinicians sometimes find it easier to schedule a series of 15-min visits, rather than one 45-min family meeting, both in terms of managing time and dealing with financial reimbursement from third-party payees. However, the clinician and family would likely benefit by convening the longer family meeting, in order to allow adequate time for exploration and discussion in the following situations [3]:

- Discussing a new diagnosis, especially if the treatment is complex
- Understanding the impact of a chronic condition on a family
- When a psychosocial problem is the main concern of the patient
- Family conflict interfering with treatment
- Dealing with any of the following: hospitalization, terminal illness, institutionalization, and death

Family Conference

As the second form of a family visit, the family-oriented clinician convenes a 30–45-min **family conference**. This is routine in any of the situations listed above, or if he or she just feels stuck about what to do next—just as liver function tests would be ordered for a jaundiced patient [3].

Think Family (with Individual Patients)

The family-oriented clinician consistently considers family context, even with individual patients. The primary care clinician who meets with individual patients most of the time can develop a family focus by integrating five family-oriented questions routinely into the 15-min office visit [21]. The patient's presenting complaint is the entry point into the family context.

> A woman with musculoskeletal pain describes difficulty with accomplishing her activities of daily living. She has problems moving early in the morning due to stiffness. The clinician uses that information to ask if she is able to solicit support from family members to help. This leads to a discussion of her husband's response to her health problems.

The five family-oriented questions are [21]:

1. Has anyone else in the family had the problem?
   Often, the answer to this question will elucidate information that directly impacts how the patient manages his or her own illness.
2. What do family members believe caused the problem and how do they believe it should be treated?
   The family's theory of illness and the meaning attributed to the illness can support or undermine effective treatment.

Clinician	Tell me your husband's understanding and ideas about your illness.
Patient	My husband thinks I need be tougher and do more for myself.

3. Who in the family is most concerned about the problem?
   This might identify family members who would be most helpful with the treatment plan, or if outside support will be needed.
4. Along with your illness, have there been any other recent changes or stresses in your life?
5. How can your family or friends be helpful to you in dealing with this problem?

These five questions can be integrated into the 15-min office visit by weaving the psychosocial questions in with the purely biomedical inquiries. The process seems natural and seamless [20].

Patient	I have a lot of pain in the morning. I have a hard time doing simple things, like the laundry.
Clinician	That sounds difficult. Who in the family is most concerned about your suffering?
Patient	That would be my daughter. She stops over to help whenever she can. My husband wants me to try to be more active. He thinks it would help if I pushed myself to do more.
Clinician	What do you think?
Patient	I don't know.
Clinician	How do you think your husband could be more helpful?
Patient	I think it would help if he understood more about my condition.
Clinician	I think it might be a good idea for you and your husband to come together for the next appointment. I find it helpful when couples talk about a medical problem together. Often, they develop better solutions than either one could figure out by him or herself.
Patient	Okay.

References

1. Kadis LB, McClendon R. Marital and family therapy. Washington, DC: American Psychiatric Press; 1998.
2. Joines V. Couples therapy. In: Kadis LB, editor. Redecision therapy: expanded perspectives. Watsonville, CO: Western Institute for Group and Family Therapy; 1985.
3. McDaniel SH, Campbell TC, Hepworth J, Lorenz A. Family-oriented primary care. 2nd ed. New York, NY: Springer; 2005.
4. Wynne LC, Singer MT. Thought disorder and family relations of schizophrenics. Arch Gen Psychiatry. 1963;9:191–8.
5. Coyne JC. Depression, biology, marriage and marital therapy. Fam Pract. 1987;13:393–407.
6. Campbell TL. The effectiveness of family interventions for physical disorder. J Marital Fam Ther. 2003;29:263–81.

7. Morisky PE, Levine DM, Green LW, Shapiro S, Russell RP, Smith CR. Five-year blood pressure and mortality following health education for hypertensive patients. Am J Public Health. 1983;73:153–62.

8. Report of the National Heart, Lung, and Blood Institute Working group. Management of patient compliance in the treatment of hypertension. Hypertension. 1982;4:415–23.

9. Bader E, Pearson P. In quest of the mythical mate: a developmental approach to diagnosis and treatment in couples therapy. Florence, KY: Brunner/Mazel; 1988.

10. Pearson P, Bader E. Couples in conflict [audio]. 2011. http://couplesinstitute.com. Accessed 10 Feb 2011.

11. Minuchin S, Montalvo B, Guerney BG, Rosmann BL, Schumer F. Families of the slums: an exploration of their structure and treatment. New York, NY: Basic Books; 1967.

12. Minuchin S. Families and family therapy. Cambridge, MA: Harvard University Press; 1974.

13. Black C. It will never happen to me. 2nd ed. Center City, MN: Hazeldon; 1987.

14. Joines V. Redecision family therapy. In: Kalson FW, Massey RF, editors. Comprehensive handbook of psychotherapy, vol. 3. Hoboken, NJ: Wiley; 2004.

15. Allmond B, Tanner J, Gofman H. The family is the patient: using family interviews in children's medical care. 2nd ed. Baltimore, MD: Williams and Williams; 1999.

16. Berne E. Games people play; the basic handbook of transactional analysis. New York, NY: Grove; 1969.

17. Carter B, McGoldrick M. Overview: the changing family cycle – a framework for family therapy. In: Carter B, McGoldrick M, editors. The changing family life cycle. 2nd ed. Boston, MA: Allyn and Bacon; 1989.

18. Hunter C, Goodie J, Oordt M, Dohmeyer A. Integrated behavioral health in primary care. Washington, DC: American Psychological Association; 2009.

19. Betancourt JR. Culture competency: providing quality care to diverse populations. Consult Pharm. 2006;21:988–95.

20. Doherty WJ, Baird MA. Family therapy and family medicine. New York, NY: The Guilford Press; 1983.

21. Cole-Kelly K, Seaburn D. Five areas of questioning to promote a family-oriented approach in primary care. Fam Syst Health. 1999;17:340–8.

Chapter 13
Family Interviewing

Role Play

It is important that the trainee beginning to participate in family role plays first learn the following individual interviewing tools: **listening**, *clarifying*, **open-ended inquiries, personal story, contracting**, *eliciting feeling*, **empathic summaries, transition statements, theory of illness, behavioral incident, affirming family members' strengths**, and **restatement** (see Chaps. 1–11).

Once the trainee has demonstrated mastery, as well as the ability to generalize the above skills to novel situations, he or she is ready to jump right into family role plays. Role plays can be created from trainee cases or created de novo. The key principles for effective role plays listed in the introduction are fully applicable with families. Typically the role plays go for 5–10 min, but a 20-min time period can be devoted to a macrotraining. Transcripts of three representative role plays follow.

Potential Role Play Objectives

1. Join with each family member
2. Avoid coalitions
3. Contract with each family member
4. Stop any interruptions and establish any necessary guidelines
5. Explore a problem adequately, but not spend too much time
6. Demonstrate circular questioning
7. Do an enactment
8. Use a transition statement when moving conversation between family members
9. List family strengths (use an easel board)
10. Set clear, specific goals collaboratively

The online version of this chapter (doi:10.1007/978-1-4614-7224-7_13) contains supplementary material, which is available to authorized users.

Role Play #1:   The Fleming family is meeting with the doctor in the hospital to discuss placement of Mr. Fleming in a long-term facility. He has late stage Alzheimer's. They have a 45-minute meeting scheduled. His son Jack, daughter-in-law, Mary, and two daughters, Stacy and Annette are present.

Objectives

1. Stop interruptions and establish guideline of one person talking at a time
2. Maintain an empathic stance with all family members

An actor, an actress, and two volunteers play the family. This role play begins with the third phase of the interview (discuss the problem).

Trainee	Stacy, will you tell us your perspective on how to deal with your dad's condition.
Stacy	I think he really has gone downhill recently. It is getting very stressful, trying to arrange 24-hour care for him. The workers have been unreliable at times and we all have had to jump in and help. I don't mind, but it is wearing us all out.
Annette	I don't think there is any choice. He needs to be placed in a facility that can give him the care that he needs. It is the best thing for dad and everyone....
Stacy	(*interrupting in a very loud voice*) I can't believe you are saying this...
Trainee	(*interrupting and putting up his hand to stop Stacy*) Let's make a rule: each person is entitled to his or her own thoughts and feelings. Will everyone agree to this and that one person talks at a time.
Family	We agree. (*Stacy is very quiet*)
Trainee	Mary or Jack, we have not heard your opinions. Will you tell your perspectives?

Feedback

Faculty	Okay. Let's stop. Affirmations?
Trainee #2	I thought you did a good job including the different family members.

(continued)

Trainee #3	I think you met your objective of stopping any interruptions and establishing necessary guidelines.
Faculty	I thought your guideline was clear. You took charge.
Trainee	Thanks.
Faculty	Does anybody have options?
Stacy	I think it would help to let me say my piece first before stating the guideline. I felt a little bit attacked.
Faculty	(*to trainee*) What do you think?
Trainee	I agree. I felt like I shut her down.
Faculty	Say more about that.
Trainee	I think I got a little anxious and jumped in too soon.
Faculty	Nice awareness. Anxiety often leads to rushing the interaction. Staying aware allows you to manage that anxiety. How might you do that?
Trainee	I could remind myself that the family conflict is not likely to get out of control and that I can intervene if it did.
Faculty	Let's run it back. During this role play, plan to let her say her piece and empathize with her position before establishing the guideline.
Trainee	Yes.

Replay

Trainee	Who would like to start off and say their perspective?
Jack	Since Mary and I live out of town, we miss a lot of what is going on. It seems to me we need a different agency. The workers frequently call in sick.
Annette	I don't know Jack. I'm not sure we can afford a better agency. Maybe we need to consider a long term facility. Dad is….
Stacy	(*interrupting*) I can't believe you are saying this. Dad….
Annette	(*interrupting*) I was just saying….
Stacy	(*interrupting in a loud voice*) Dad would never want that. He would rather die.
Trainee	Stacy, it sounds like you value highly what your dad would have wanted.
Stacy	Of course. It is the least he deserves.
Trainee	I would like to propose a guideline. You all have important things to say. It has been my experience that folks are better able to listen to one another when one person talks at a time and each person's opinion is respected. Is that okay?
Family	Of course.

Feedback

Faculty	Good job. You had a nice expression of empathy and established the guideline. It seemed warm. How did it feel to you Stacy?
Stacy	I felt heard.

Role Play #2: Mr. and Mrs. Green have come for a consultation about the treatment of their son for ADHD. Workup and discussion of ADHD was recently completed, and they wanted time to think about treatment recommendations.

Objective

Spend time hearing each person's perspective on the problem, but not too much time on any one person.

Trainee	Hi Mr. and Mrs. Green. It is good to see you again. We agreed to talk, today, about treatment for Travis's ADHD. Who wants to start and tell me what your ideas are about treatment?
Mother	I'll start. I think he needs medicine. I'm the one who is with him 24 hours a day. Tom, I know you don't agree but you don't see what I see. He sits and fidgets for an hour without getting any homework done. It is so frustrating. I don't think he can help it. His backpack is a mess. Papers everywhere. The morning is a disaster. If I didn't help him, he never would make it on time. I don't have to help his sister—she is sitting ready to go. I am afraid that if something does not change soon, Travis will be left further and further behind. I don't want him on medication if it is not necessary, but I think he really needs it. Jennifer says it helped Joseph a lot.
Trainee	Mrs. Green, let me jump in here for a second. You are very concerned about Travis because you are with him 24 hours a day. You see him struggling with being disorganized and distractible. It is affecting him every day, and you think he might need medication, even though you wished he didn't need it. Is that right?
Mother	Yes.
Trainee	Mr. Green, What do you think?

(continued)

Father	I don't think using medicine is a good idea. I have read how they are being overprescribed. I was just like Travis when I was his age and I did okay. Aren't there some other things we can do, Doc?
Trainee	Well, there are some other interventions we can discuss. However, the evidence shows they don't work as well.
Father	Maybe, they would work for Travis

Feedback

Faculty	Let me stop it here. (*to trainee*) First, what do you like about your interview?
Trainee	I thought I didn't get flustered and I kept them on track.
Faculty	You did. Anybody have other affirmations.
Trainee #2	I thought you (*trainee*) did a good job, especially letting Mrs. Green talk without interrupting her.
Trainee #3	I liked your empathy with Mrs. Green. You listened to her concerns and then summarized them back to her.
Mother	I did feel you listened to what it was like for me.
Faculty	Anybody have options?
Father	I thought you wanted me to agree to medication and I didn't want to use them.
Faculty	(*to trainee*) What do you think?
Trainee	I see his point. I did think Travis should be on medication.
Faculty	The father might be more willing to hear your recommendation after you explore his concerns in more depth. He may have a misperception about stimulants that you could resolve. Why don't you replay from the point he says he does not think medication is a good idea. The primary objective will be to understand father's perspective.
Trainee	Okay. I'll try to understand his view better.

Replay

Father	I don't know if medication is a good idea. I have read where they are being overprescribed.
Trainee	Tell me more about your concern.

(continued)

Father	I know Ritalin is a classified drug. I've read that high school and college kids sell it. I don't want to put my child on a medicine that is going to make him a zombie.
Trainee	So, you believe that Travis will not be himself on the medicine. In addition, you have read how older kids sell it to other kids because of its powerful effects. No wonder you are concerned. Would it be okay if we discuss this further?
Father	Yes.
Faculty	Let's stop. You used a gentle command, "Tell me more about your concerns," and the father talked. You are in a better position to understand and address his concerns now.

Macrotraining

Role Play #3:   A 54-year-old man is in for follow up of a mild MI experienced 4 weeks ago. He is accompanied by his wife of 28 years. The clinician requested he bring her for this visit because of the clinician's concerns regarding his cardiac rehabilitation and overall adjustment (16–17 minutes into the interview)

Objective

Structure a 20-min routine office visit with the five-phase outline, staying within the time limits and establishing a plan of action

Patient	I don't go to rehab because I feel fine.
Trainee	What do you mean?
Patient	I feel good. I take my medicines religiously. I don't really have time to go to rehab. I wish my wife would just let me decide for myself.
Trainee	Mrs. Miller, what are you feeling when your husband says this?
Patient	I can't help worrying. I don't want it to happen again, or even be worse next time. It was really frightening for me. (*eyes fill up with tears momentarily*)
Trainee	I can imagine. If you picture something worse next time, no wonder you worry. We will have to do some education about recovery

(continued)

from a heart attack. It might also be helpful for you to learn ways
of managing your anxiety so that you feel more relaxed.

Wife   Okay.

(later in the interview)

Trainee   Let me see if I have this right: Mr. Miller you feel you are doing
well. You are able to work full time. Mrs. Miller, you are worried
that he is right back to overworking. You main worry is that he
might have another heart attack. So you try to get him to go rehab.
It helped your brother-in-law recover from a similar heart attack.
In addition, you worry about your husband's cholesterol level and
encourage him to eat more healthily. Only, it doesn't work because,
Mr. Miller, you feel she is hovering. You then pull away. Mrs.
Miller, you respond by getting even more anxious and remind your
husband about his diet and going to rehab. Is that right?

Wife   Exactly. Let me tell you what happened this weekend. I made a
low fat dinner and he didn't eat it, but then he had ice cream after
dinner... (*5 minutes later*) ... I want to help him if he would just
let me.

Faculty   We are almost out of time, so please wrap up.

Trainee   Well, Mr. and Mrs. Miller will you agree to an experiment? For the
next 2 weeks, Mrs. Miller, don't remind him about eating well or
going to rehab. When you return, we can discuss cardiac rehabilitation, again. How does that sound?

Patient   Okay.

Wife   I will do my best if it would help.

Feedback

Faculty   (*to trainee*) Tell what you like about what you did.

Trainee   I engaged both people in the family. I organized the interview.
I felt rushed at the end.

Faculty   We will get to that in a second. First let's go over what you did well.
I wrote a number of positive interventions all along the way. You got
a clear contract at the beginning from each person. You joined with
both Mr. and Mrs. Miller. I like the way you invited Mrs. Miller to
tell her personal story. You gave her lots of space to talk. You heard
both people's perspectives and elicited their feelings. I liked the

(continued)

way you used empathic summaries to acknowledge their feelings, as well as to transition between the phases of the interview smoothly. I think your assessment of the couple dynamics is accurate. I do have one or two options. Are you ready to hear them?

Trainee   Sure

Faculty   Manage your time to allow 5–6 minutes at the end to identify their strengths and develop a plan. It would have been easier to collaborate with them on a plan, rather than just giving it to them. They are likely to own the plan if it comes from them. I would suggest limiting the discussion of the problem to 7–10 minutes. I think you can hear enough of the story in that time to understand the problem. They do have real strengths upon which you can draw. They care about each other deeply, and have managed a number of stresses in the past with their grown children. Does that make sense to you?

Trainee   Definitely. I did feel I was just telling them what to do, instead of collaborating. I think discussing the problem long enough to understand it, but also limiting the discussion, will help.

Trainee   Let's replay it starting from the summary you gave to Mr. and Mrs. Miller.

Replay

Trainee   Let me see if I have this right: Mr. Miller you feel you are doing well. You are able to work full time. Mrs. Miller, you are worried that he is right back to overworking. You main worry is that he might have another heart attack. So you try to get him to eat healthy and go to rehab. Only, it doesn't work because Mr. Miller, you feel she is hovering. You then pull away. Mrs. Miller, you respond by getting even more anxious and remind your husband about his diet and going to rehab. Is that right?

Wife   That's it. It is very frustrating. Just last weekend I baked a fish dinner. He wouldn't eat it. Instead, he ate several bowls of ice cream after dinner. If I say anything he gets angry.

Trainee   Let me step in here for a minute. I hear how frustrating this has been for you. In terms of time, I would like to leave enough time to develop a plan of action. We can meet again, since it is clear we haven't fully finished with this issue.

(continued)

Wife	Sure.
Trainee	Before we develop a specific plan, tell me about your personal strengths and resources. I think that will help us in planning.
Wife	We have a solid marriage of 28 years and we have two grown children who would help out if we asked.
Patient	We have worked hard all our life.
Trainee	So, you are resourceful people.
Patient	Yes.
Trainee	Would you both tell me what you think would work best for you as a family?
Patient	I would like to try a period of time where I am not reminded about how I should eat or whether I should go to rehab.
Trainee	That is about what you would like your wife to do. Are there any changes you would be willing to make to take care of your own health?
Patient	I would be willing to discuss a diet with my wife and stick with it for the most part, as long as she doesn't remind me.
Trainee	Would you be willing to stick with the diet even if she reminds you.
Patient	(*laughs*) I guess so.
Wife	(*to husband*) I see how my reminders bother you. I don't want to be like that.
Trainee	Nice awareness. It will be important for you to learn strategies to manage your anxiety.
Wife	Yes.
Trainee	What about rehab, Mr. Miller.
Patient	I would like more time to think about that.
Faculty	Okay. Let's stop. Good job. You got the message.

Obstacles to Family Role Plays

1. Interviewer doesn't understand the importance of involving family to improve patient health outcomes.
2. Interviewer lacks experience and confidence.
3. Interviewer is concerned it will take too much time.
4. Trainee believes that it would be too difficult to get real families to come in for a meeting.
5. Trainee avoids certain family situations because of resemblance to own family.

Strategies

1. Educate trainees about the impact of families on individual health.
2. Practice and master skills in this book via role plays. Go for extra training. Contract for supervision of cases with a qualified family therapist.
3. Acknowledge it can take a few extra minutes to see families during routine office visits initially. Later, it may actually take less time.
4. Teach trainees skills for closing excursions into discussing family issues during office visits with individual patients (see "closing the window" in Chap. 7).
5. Teach skills for dealing with resistance (e.g., not debating, listening, frame meeting as a way to help patient, call family members directly).
6. Use a group format to deal with "issues in the clinician."

Family Interviewing[1]

Family interviewers meet with families in a variety of circumstances. They might see an elderly couple together in an informal office visit, talk briefly to family members gathered at a patient's bedside, or conduct a planned family conference for a family contemplating hospice care for their father. In all these circumstances, the clinician must structure the visit in terms of time and communication flow. He or she must direct traffic. The family is a group, and as a group, they can present all kinds of new challenges to the interviewer. Family members might talk over one another, argue, remain silent but agitated, or even invite the clinician to take sides. The family clinician must take charge of the meeting. This demands a different type of leadership from that required with individual patients.

The family-oriented clinician is faced with the task of mastering new skills and adapting his or her individual interviewing skills to a group format. **These core family interviewing skills can be categorized into five general areas, corresponding to the phases of the interview suggested by McDaniel et al. [1]. The principles are applicable to both routine 20-min office visits and prearranged 30–45-min family conferences.**

Rapport

It is important to make the first priority joining with each member of the family, and not move on until **rapport** has been established [1]. The clinician asks each family member for his or her personal story. Generally, each person takes 1–2 min to tell

[1]The structure for a family meeting is adapted from Family-Oriented Primary Care, 2nd edn. McDaniel, Campbell, Hepworth and Lorenz with permission, Springer, 2012.

his or her personal story. A safe atmosphere to talk freely is established by affirming each person's strengths, listening carefully, and tracking with each person. It can be a challenge to listen and acknowledge each person's distressed feelings in a large family. In terms of generating trust in the clinician and a sense of hopefulness about the possibility of change, the dividends are enormous [2]. Tanner and Allmond label this process as **touching** the family members.

Simultaneously, the clinician is attuned to what is going on in the family at the process level. The clinician wants to accommodate to the family personality and communication style by matching his or her responses to the tone and nonverbal behavior of the family [2]. To calm an anxious family, the clinician might adopt a soft but firm voice and a slow pace. Thought-provoking questions and comments would help initiate contact with an intellectualizing family, while playful responses would mirror the presentation of a boisterous family. When a family and a clinician have major difference in terms of age, gender, race, ethnicity, and socioeconomic status, it is especially important for the clinician to find a **common language** to join with the family [1]. In the following exchange of dialogue, a nurse enters the exam room of an 8-year-old boy and his family. She engages with the family by attending to heritage.

Nurse	Johnny, I see you have a shamrock on your shirt
Johnny	My grandparents gave it to me. They got it in Ireland.
Nurse	How neat.
Mother	Would you like to see pictures of the visit?
Nurse	I sure would.
Mother	This is my parents taking a traditional carriage ride. My dad was born in Ireland and this was his only trip back.
Nurse	They must have had a wonderful time.
Mother	It was like magic. Look at the smiles on their faces while taking the carriage ride. Of course, my dad felt sad leaving his relatives at the end of the trip.
Nurse	You know, my parents are from Romania. They miss their family terribly. I can really appreciate how much that visit must have meant to your parents and to you.

The astute clinician is careful to join with each family member, avoiding invitations to form a coalition against another family member. The clinician declines any invitation to take sides by pointing out that everyone's opinion is valued, and, in fact, he or she will better be able to help the patient by understanding the problem more fully [1].

Daughter	Doctor, will you agree with me that my husband should set a good example for Johnny?
Clinician	Mrs. Jones, I want to hear your ideas and concerns, as well as understand the thoughts of both your husband and Johnny, before we discuss what would be the best option for helping Johnny with his weight. It will be important to have all this information, so you as a family can make the best choice about how to deal with this problem.

Organize/Contract

Leadership of a family session is established by taking charge of the session, structuring, and setting guidelines [2]. It starts with the first contact with the family. A high value is placed on family involvement. The clinician does not accept a patient's initial response that the family cannot or will not come to an office visit or family meeting [1]. The clinician listens and empathizes with any challenges of setting up a meeting. Persisting, the clinician states that the family members are needed to help him or her help the patient. The **family is not asked to attend a meeting because of a family problem**, which can lead to defensiveness. Most families will agree to a meeting in order to help another family member [1].

The family-oriented clinician sets the tone for the visit by modeling respect for each person and directing the flow smoothly through the phases of the interview. The session begins and ends on time. He or she conveys a sense of confidence that the family can cope with an illness or solve a problem.

The exam room is organized so people can sit and see each other as they talk. Crayons and paper, set out for the younger children, can keep them occupied during the meeting. If children are misbehaving and interfering with the meeting, the clinician might ask the parents to get the children under control (if parents are capable), or have an adult watch the children outside the exam room.

Once the family members are in the room and the clinician has joined with them, a contract for the visit is established. **An agreement to a clear contract for the family session is an essential preliminary step to being able to understand and help a family with an illness or problem.** Sometimes, contracting is straightforward: *We plan to meet for 45 min to look for solutions to manage your mother's decreased ability to care for herself.* Even then, the contact may need to be renegotiated as more information about the situation and family dynamics becomes available. On many occasions, a clinician must persist in asking family members to explain and clarify, until a specific, doable agreement is reached. If family members repeatedly interrupt each other during this process, the clinician will ask them for an agreement that one person talk at a time [2]. In the following dialogue, the clinician works to obtain an agreement about the next step forward for excessive weight gain identified during an 8-year-old well child visit.

Clinician	Looking at the growth curve, I notice that Johnny's weight increased significantly more than his height in the last year. Have you noticed this also?
Mother	Yes. I have encouraged him to play outside more.
Clinician	Is this an issue you would be willing to discuss?
Mother	Sure
Father	Okay.
Clinician	Before we start discussing what to do about the situation, I would like to get clear about the different aspects of the issue.
Mother	Most of my family members are large people. He may just have unlucky genes.
Father	(*remains quiet*)
Trainee	Mr. Jones, I notice you have not said anything yet. What do you think?
Father	My wife is probably correct. Her family is large. Also, he doesn't have many friends to play with in our neighborhood, so he mostly has to watch television and play video games.
Clinician	Johnny, what do you think about all this?
Johnny	I do like to play outside. Sometimes, I have nobody to play with.
Mother	We live out in the country.
Clinician	Let me see if I have it correct so far… All three of you think it would be a good idea for Johnny to be more active.
Parents	Yes.
Clinician	I think I may have jumped a step ahead of myself. I would like to back up for a second. Do you see the increased weight gain as an important problem?
Parents	Yes.
Clinician	How about you Johnny?
Johnny	I guess.
Clinician	Sometimes, children tell me it is a problem. They get teased about their weight. Has that happened at your school?
Johnny	One kid does call me names.
Clinician	What has that been like for you?
Johnny	I just ignore him.
Clinician	That sounds like a smart idea. Do you feel sad or mad about what he says?
Johnny	A little sad.
Clinician	I think any kid would feel that way. Let me see if I understand everything so far… As a family, you all want Johnny to be more active. You see the weight gain as a problem. It sounds like it is an important issue to all of you. It is good that you all are involved, since a change of this magnitude does take each mem-

(continued)

	ber of the family making an individual commitment to change him or herself.
Parents	We want to help Johnny in any way we can.
Clinician	It is a complex issue and there are many aspects. We will need to discuss what contributes to a healthy weight, such as hereditary, exercise, eating habits, and even how feelings are dealt with in the family. We will also talk about what families generally do about this type of problem, and what you, as a family think would work best for your particular family. How about we set aside a time to discuss this more fully in the next 1–2 weeks?
Parents	Okay.
Clinician	How does that sound to you Johnny?
Johnny	It's okay with me too.

Facilitate Discussion and Transmit Information

Discussion of the problem is the core of phase three, which occurs once the engagement is solid and a clear contract for the meeting has been established. The perspective of family members is solicited. The clinician includes everyone. Conversely, no one family member is allowed to monopolize. Passive members are invited to participate:

Patient	(*not participating*)
Clinician	Mr. Jones, it would really help me to hear your ideas. Your perspective is important in order for us to figure out the best way to solve this problem.

Inquiring into the perspectives of other family members may introduce new medical data. **The clinician will want to learn about the family's understanding of the patient's illness, the meaning they have placed on the illness, how it has affected them, and what they have already done about it**. It is important to hear enough about the problem from a family member's perspective, and leave time to hear the perspective of others.

Johnny's mother talks about the specifics of his overeating. She connects the origins of his problem to his early life experiences. The clinician listens carefully. He then moves the discussion to another family member, transitioning with an introduced gate:

Mother	My mother died the year Johnny was born. I probably have given Johnny extra slack with limits, including eating habits, because he is an only child and his grandmother passed. She would have been a wonderful grandmother.
Clinician	It sounds like a big loss for you and him. (*silence*) I would like to move to Johnny now. We have not yet heard his thoughts about his weight. (*introduced gate*)

Several techniques can be utilized to clarify the relationship dynamics, which may be contributing to the medical condition. In addition, the medical condition very well may be impacting family relationships. Ways to assess this information include:

1. Asking for a recent, specific example of the situation; track the reaction of the family (see **behavioral incident** in Chap. 7)
2. Use **circular questioning**
3. Set up an **enactment**

Circular questioning is a style of interviewing designed to uncover information about differences or changes in relationships that have occurred as a result of an illness or problem [3]. It is a clever and powerful tool. Once learned, it is easy to use. The following, brief dialogue with a couple utilizes circular questioning to make their underlying process clear. In other instances, an interviewer might ask one family member to comment on the differences he or she has observed in the interactions of other family members as a result of a problem.

Mother	Johnny is a good kid. I don't think it would be fair to restrict his food intake.
Clinician	What are you feeling as you think that?
Mother	I feel sad.
Clinician	What's goes on inside you, Joe, when you hear about your wife's sadness.
Father	I feel bad. I'm not sure a diet is necessary.
Clinician	So, Joe, when you see your wife sad how do you respond behaviorally?
Father	I usually try to help her not feel sad.
Clinician	How do you do that?
Father	I make a joke—try to jolly her out of it.
Clinician	Rebecca, when Joe does that, how do you react?
Mother	I usually pretend I'm not sad. We don't really talk about negative stuff.

(continued)

Clinician	Joe, it sounds like it is difficult to see your wife feeling sad.
Father	We are all like that. None of us want to see anyone in the family feeling badly.
Clinician	Is that true for you too Johnny?
Johnny	I guess.

An *enactment* involves two or more family members talking to each other about a situation or problem [4]. This interaction occurs "in the room," allowing the clinician the opportunity to observe, firsthand, family patterns of communication and relating. The family is literally showing the clinician their process. The enactment is set up by telling the participants to face each other and talk about a topic for a specified time period. The clinician places his or her chair away from the dialogue and observes. If a participant turns to the clinician to talk, the clinician simply replies: *Tell it to him (or her)* .... One key to handling this type of resistance is to encourage the participants to continue to talk to each other [5].

Clinician	Would you be willing to talk with each other about the problem? It seems that you have different ideas about how to help your son. Talk to each other as if I were not present.
Parents	We have already done that at home.
Clinician	Would you do it anyway?
Parents	Okay.

Bader and Pearson suggest watching each participant's ability to do the following tasks as a way of assessing their developmental level [6]:

- Listen carefully
- Acknowledge and accept the feelings of the other
- Stick to one topic
- Express his or her thinking and feelings clearly
- Not attack the other

It would be unwise to set upon enactment with a very hostile or violent couple.

Identify Strengths, Resources, and Supports

Family members adapt best to chronic illness and make lifestyle changes when they view themselves from an okay position, from an "I can do this" position. Helping a family identify their strengths and resources encourages them to take an active stance in relation to the patient's illness. This helps avoid the use of less effective resources outside the family [1]. One way to encourage a family to recognize and acknowledge their strengths is to brainstorm with the family, listing them on an easel board [1]. In the following dialogue, Johnny and his parents list their strengths.

Clinician	I would like to move to get a good handle on your strengths and resources before we develop a plan. Why don't I list them on the easel board, so we can keep track of them.
Mother	Well, we have been happily married for 15 years. I think that's a big plus.
Clinician	I agree. So let's put a strong, committed marriage. What else?
Father	I am not sure what to say.
Clinician	Mr. Jones, I have known you a long time. I know you are not the type to blow your own horn. The point of this exercise is to list all your resources in order to help you deal with this problem.
Mother	Doctor, you know we have been through a lot. We don't give up.
Clinician	So let's put down a resourceful and determined family.
Mother	I have two sisters who care very much about Johnny and us.
Father	We have a strong faith.
Clinician	Johnny, what do you think is the best thing about your family?
Johnny	My parents love me.
Clinician	Great. I would also like to tell you about a resource in the community that has helped a lot of the families with this exact problem....

Establish a Plan

Based on the discussion phase and subsequent formulation of the problem, the family and clinician agree to a treatment plan that will help move them in a positive direction and to a new contract. This may include psychoeducation, the development of specific, concrete goals, or a family therapy referral.

The clinician states the plan clearly: *Johnny, Mr. and Mrs. Jones, you all agree to return in the next 2 weeks for a 30-minute visit to explore options for helping*

Johnny with his weight. He or she checks in with each person for understanding and agreement with the treatment plan. When family members do not agree to a common ground and problems persist, arrangements for a mental health referral are made.

Key Points

1. A five-part sequence can be used to structure routine office family visits and longer family conferences.
2. The five phases are:

   - Rapport
   - Organize/contract
   - Facilitate discussion and transmit information
   - Identify strengths, resources and supports
   - Establish a plan

3. Each phase of the family interview has specific tasks and goals.
4. It is important to manage time so that all phases of the interview are allocated sufficient time.

References

1. McDaniel SH, Campbell TC, Hepworth J, Lorenz A. Family-oriented primary care. 2nd ed. New York, NY: Springer; 2005.
2. Allmond B, Tanner J, Gofman H. The family is the patient: using family interviews in children's medical care. 2nd ed. Baltimore, MD: Williams and Wilkins; 1999.
3. Penn P. Circular questioning. Fam Process. 1982;21:267–80.
4. Minuchin S, Fishman H. Family therapy techniques. Cambridge, MA: Harvard University Press; 1981.
5. Nichols M, Fellenberg S. The effective use of enactments in family therapy: a discovery-oriented process study. J Marital Fam Ther. 2000;26:143–52.
6. Bader E, Pearson P. In quest of the mythical mate: a developmental approach to diagnoses and treatment in couples therapy. Florence, KY: Brunner/Mazel; 1988.

Chapter 14
Mental Health

Role Play

The following role play assumes mastery of core interviewing skills (Chaps. 1–11), as well as focused questioning, which is needed for making specific diagnoses.

Role Play: A 42-year-old man has intermittent low back pain, but has been otherwise well. He is a lawyer in a busy practice. His chief complaint is insomnia.

Objective (12–15-min Role Play)

Fully assess depression region (screen for neurovegetative symptoms, including suicidality; check out medical and substance abuse causes; psychosocial history; psychiatric history of patient and family)

Trainee	Mr. Evans, insomnia can be caused by a wide variety of conditions, including sleep apnea, pain, stress and depression. I am going to ask you about all that. Is that ok.
Patient	Well I have been stressed at work. I recently lost a couple of important clients. It has been weighing on my mind a lot.
Trainee	Let me start by asking two questions. Over the last two weeks, have you felt down, depressed, or hopeless?
Patient	No, I have been very anxious though.
Trainee	Over the last two weeks have you felt little pleasure in doing things?

(continued)

J. Binder, *Primary Care Interviewing: Learning Through Role Play*,
DOI 10.1007/978-1-4614-7224-7_14, © Springer Science+Business Media New York 2013

Patient	Yes. I agree with that statement.
Trainee	Tell me all about your lack of pleasure in doing thing. Start at the beginning and walk me through it.
Patient	I started having problems 3–4 months ago, when I had a couple of bad outcomes with clients. I started staying later to deal with my cases. I have even stayed all night in the office several times recently. My wife is concerned about me. I feel guilty about not being home much, but I don't feel I have a choice. I think I could lose my job.
Trainee	Let me see if I have this right. You are very anxious about your work since you had some unfortunate outcomes with clients. You are overworking and your wife is concerned about you as a result. Is that it?
Patient	That's it.
Trainee	I would like to ask you some specific questions about how this has affected you? You said it has affected your sleep. How has it affected sleep?

The trainee then guides the patient through the neurovegetative symptoms.

Trainee	Let me summarize what you have said do far… You have been stressed and anxious for several months and have felt down the last three weeks. You are feeling very guilty about several mistakes you made at work. You are sleeping 4–5 hours a night, and you don't feel yourself at all. Your sex drive is down. You have withdrawn socially and stopped exercising. You have gained close to 10 pounds. You have really been suffering.
Patient	Yea. I have felt like I am in a dark place.
Trainee	Lots of people have thoughts of suicide when they get to feeling so down. Has that been true of you?
Patient	No, I have thought about death, but not suicide.
Trainee	Tell me more.
Patient	I don't think of killing myself. I want to live. I just want to feel better.
Trainee	Of course… Mr. Evans, have you ever had a period of time when you were feeling the opposite of what you are now—when you were feeling hyper, and people thought you were not yourself?
Patient	No, but my mom did. She was diagnosed with manic depression and was hospitalized several times when I was a kid. She would lose touch with reality.

(continued)

Trainee	Anybody else with bipolar depression or others types of depression?
Patient	No.
Trainee	I have a couple more questions. Have you had any serious medical problems?
Patient	None.
Trainee	Are you on any medications?
Patient	No.
Trainee	Ok, I think that is it.

Feedback

Faculty	Great job. You structured the interview very well. I liked your pace. You had a solid engagement all along. I thought you used summaries well, both to empathize and to guide the interview. You covered all the neurovegetative symptoms. You asked about medical problems, medication, and considered bipolar depression as part of your differential. You asked about suicide after you had set the platform and it seemed very natural. Mr. Evans, how did it feel being the patient?
Patient	Wonderful. I felt you (*trainee*) cared. You took your time and listened carefully to me. Also I felt like you knew what you were doing, by the way you moved through the questions.
Faculty	Say more about the way the clinician asked the questions.
Patient	I noticed that you summarized the history several times, and then moved the interview to specific symptoms I hadn't mentioned. It seemed like you had a plan. This gave me confidence you were knowledgeable and would be able to help me.
Faculty	That is an important reason to structure the interview. If this were a real situation, you would also perform a mental status exam and physical exam. I do have one option. That is to ask about alcohol and drug abuse. That is an important differential.
Trainee	I thought of it earlier and forgot to come back to it.
Faculty	One thing I do when I think of something, but it is not a good time to ask about it, is to jot it down on a piece of paper as a reminder to return to it later in the interview.

Obstacles to Assessing and Treatment of Mental Health Conditions During Training

1. Interviewer lacks expert mentoring during training, diagnosing, and treating mental health conditions.
2. There is a lack of priority given to mental conditions in terms of teaching time.
3. Interviewer fears becoming overwhelmed with the emotions of patients.
4. Use of the biomedical model is widespread and entrenched in medicine.
5. Clinician depletion.

Strategies

1. Learn on the job as part of a team, with medical psychologist acting as expert consultant and teacher.
2. Demonstrate to trainees the ability to stay emotionally present to a patient expressing feelings.
3. Teach closing skills (structuring tools) when dealing with emotions.
4. Show evidence to trainees that the biopsychosocial model is evidence-based.
5. Promote clinician self-care (Balint-type groups; retreats).

Mental Health

The number of patients receiving treatment for mental health conditions in primary care has tripled during the last two decades [1]. Approximately one-quarter of patients in primary care present with mental health disorders [2]. In fact, all medical conditions—diabetes mellitus, COPD, depression, etc.—have both body and mind elements when viewed from a biopsychosocial model. Many chronic conditions in primary care result from lifestyle addictions, such as overeating, smoking, and drinking. Depression, anxiety, and insomnia commonly accompany those chronic illnesses [3]. In addition, virtually all primary care patients can benefit from psycho-education. A clinician in primary care must be knowledgeable of mind–body inter-actions [3]. He or she must see everyone in a limited amount of time. It is a huge demand that leaves more than 50 % of patients with emotional and mental health concerns under diagnosed and under treated [4]. A primary care clinician possess-ing the skills to engage individual patients and families, form partnerships with patients and families, structure interviews, and focus on practical concerns is in a strong position to change that statistic [4]. We will discuss the importance of these core interviewing skills in providing competent mental health assessment and treat-ment in primary care, and then transition to the interviewing skills needed to make categorical diagnoses, such as major depression.

Every primary care clinician faces two interviewing tasks:

1. Identify emotional and mental health concerns in primary care, which are often hidden from the clinician.
2. Formulate a good working diagnosis for common mental health problems.

Identifying Mental Health Disorders

Adult patients may visit the clinician multiple times before being diagnosed, or remain undiagnosed, with anxiety and depressive disorders [5, 6]. Children with anxiety or depression might not reveal their symptoms because they have trouble putting into words what they are experiencing, feel frightened, or are unaware that treatment is needed [7]. Some practices screen all their patients for psychosocial problems because they are so often hidden. Reliable and valid screens exist for both pediatric and adult patients [8, 9]. Screening all patients in a practice identifies many more people with psychosocial disorders than does surveillance (routine observation during an office visit). Practitioners who screen must develop a system of tracking the responses, evaluating positive screens, and treating or referring outliers appropriately. Whether a clinician uses screening or surveillance, he or she needs to know how to ask patients and families about mental health conditions.

Studies of physician interviewing and relationship skills have identified the key components required to identify potentially hidden emotional and mental health conditions [10, 11]. In addition, scientific evidence supports the concept that good relationship skills actually begin the treatment of mental health conditions, and are sometimes all that is needed [12]. Many people have significant problems with functioning but do not meet diagnostic criteria for a specific mental illness [13]. They can often be helped without ever making a specific diagnosis, using core interviewing skills [12].

Core Interviewing Skills

1. Engaging solidly with patients
2. Forming a true partnership
3. Structuring the visit so the focus is on practical concerns and managing any obstacles to treatment

These are the very skills we covered in the first half of this text (see Chaps. 1–7 for review). The patient must feel the emotional safety to discuss vulnerable personal issues with the clinician. A nonjudgmental attitude, caring nonverbal communication (gentle voice, slow pace, warmth, and good eye contact), open-ended inquiries, careful listening, facilitatory gestures, affirmations, eliciting feelings, and empathic reflections all contribute to emotional safety. These basic techniques encourage patients to be open and solidly engage with the clinician. A strong engagement is necessary but not sufficient to establish emotional safety.

Patients must experience the physician–patient relationship as a partnership, one in which their feelings and wishes are given equal weight with the clinician's agenda. An agreement on a clear contract for the ongoing partnership must be made explicit:

Clinician	As your doctor, I am interested in your overall health. I am not only interested in helping you with things like sore throats or rashes, but also any periods of feeling stressed and down in the dumps. In addition, I want to promote your general good health, so I plan to ask you about high risk behaviors that could impact your health. Is this all okay with you?
Patient	Yes, I am also interested in keeping myself healthy.

Specific contracts are also needed for each visit.

Clinician	I know we were going to follow up on your hypertension, today. What else would you like to put on our agenda?
Patient	My daughter and children are now living with me. I'm sure my blood pressure must be affected by that.
Clinician	Anything else for today?
Patient	That's it.

Within the context of a strong engagement, the clinician must structure the visit so that time is used efficiently to accomplish the goals set forth in the contracting process. One of the most helpful structuring tools is the empathic summary. It allows the clinician to explore and discuss an emotional topic and smoothly move back to other problems.

Clinician	Let me see if I am hearing you accurately. Your daughter moved back in with you. You want to be supportive of her, but you think she is drinking too much and taking advantage of you. You feel anxious, and are having trouble sleeping. You plan on going to Alanon, which might give you support in this tough situation. In addition, your blood pressure is up today. Given the new stresses you are facing, I would like to check out how well you have been sticking to the treatment approach we agreed to last visit.
Patient	Not so well.

One frequent and important advantage of developing structuring skills is growth in clinician confidence that he or she can handle exploration of emotional topics. A clinician's confidence in his or her mental health treatment skills leads to increased identification and discussion of emotional problems [14]. Sometimes, patients present with focused concerns or a symptom, such as sadness, and the clinician must assess for a specific diagnosis (e.g., major depression and suicidality) [4]. This requires a different set of interviewing skills.

Interview Skills Needed to Formulate a Good Differential Diagnosis

Diagnosing and treating common mental health conditions, like depression, present a real challenge to primary care clinicians. Clinical depression must be distinguished from brief situational sadness, as well as physical and psychological conditions that can mimic clinical depression [7]. A number of diagnostic questions must be answered:

- Are criteria for a specific psychiatric diagnosis met?
- Are comorbid conditions complicating the clinical picture?
- How is the patient's functioning impacted?
- What is the connection of the patient's symptoms to family functioning?
- Does the patient need a referral to a specialist?

Depression must be as thoroughly assessed as pneumonia or heart failure. If the clinician does not take a careful history, misdiagnosis can occur, such as a substance-induced mood disorder, secondary to opiate abuse, being mislabeled as major depression, resulting in inadequate treatment.

A skilled interviewer must have an organized plan—a way to differentiate clinical conditions. We saw such a plan back in Chap. 9, on the history of present illness. Only then, we were looking at mostly physical conditions like pneumonia. Symptom descriptors, such as chronology and severity, still need to be determined. In addition, the primary care clinician must know the characteristics of mental conditions and distinguish them from other mental or physical conditions. The clinician can access a range of interviewing tools to help in the process. The following series of focused questions, pulled from one questionnaire, is an example of an attempt to differentiate bipolar from unipolar depression [15].

Has there ever been a period of time when you were not your usual self and:

1. You felt so good or so hyper that other people thought you were not your normal self, or you were so hyper that you got into trouble?
2. You were so irritable that you shouted at people or started fights or arguments?
3. You felt much more self-confident than usual?

Despite the availability of a multitude of similar and helpful interviewing tools, the diagnosis of mental conditions can be complex and take considerable skill and experience. Psychiatric conditions present with both somatic and psychological manifestations, reflecting the underlying mechanisms affected by the illness. For example, the neurovegetative symptoms of a major depression derive from hypothalamic involvement, while a personal sense of unworthiness and inadequacy relate to underlying cognitive factors [16]. Therefore, inquiries regarding psychological and behavioral features are an important part of the history. The family environment and family psychiatric history take on increased importance. The family can ameliorate or conversely contribute to the illness (see Chaps. 12 and 13). The training needed to be able to formulate good working mental health diagnoses in primary care thus fall into two categories:

1. Acquire knowledge of the common mental health conditions in primary care.
2. Learn focused questions that help differentiate conditions, and consider the bio-psychosocial context.

Primary care training programs have placed more emphasis in recent years on teaching the complexity of mental health diagnosis and treatment. However, clinicians continue to feel inadequately trained [17, 18].

Collaborative Family Health Care Model

One model for providing ongoing training and good medical care at the same time is the Collaborative Family Health Care Model. This model was created to meet the heavy burden of mental healthcare needs in primary care. A psychologist operating in the primary care setting treats patients, refers patients needing specialty care, and helps promote a healthy functioning team [3]. In addition this expert acts as a consultant to the primary care clinician, a source of lifetime learning regarding mental health diagnosis and treatment.

> John is a 58–year-old male with COPD who has had infrequent episodes of respiratory distress. He was admitted to the hospital briefly with an exacerbation last winter. He smoked one pack of cigarettes a day for 32 years, quitting eight yrs. ago. He worked in construction for years. He is retired and spends his days helping his wife babysit their two young grandchildren. During his visit today he says he has been getting short of breath and is using his inhalers more frequently. He denies increased cough or sputum production during these episodes. He has had no change in appetite or sleep patterns. His exam and pulmonary function testing are unchanged. He tells the resident the shortness of breath episodes don't seem to improve when he takes his inhaler, but just resolve over time. He also reports that he is doing significantly less physical activity. The resident curbside consults the behavior psychologist, "John has become much less physically active despite an unchanged pulmonary status. Do you think John is depressed or anxious?" The psychologist has 20 minutes free and evaluates John. She diagnoses him with anxiety secondary to a medical illness, and spends time teaching him about the dyspnea/deconditioning/anxiety cycle [19], and how to manage it. She plans to see him again in two weeks to evaluate her intervention. She discussed her findings with the resident and affirms her for the referral. The resident wonders why the patient said he wasn't anxious when she asked him earlier. The psychologist takes a minute to teach the resident how some people don't recognize anxious feelings, but report anxious cognitions and avoidance behaviors when they are asked to describe a concrete, specific example of the problem situation. She agrees to discuss the assessment of anxiety, complicating a medical condition, at their weekly collaborative seminar.

This trainee learned a fact about assessing anxiety and is well positioned to improve her management of emotional and mental health issues. For example, she might be able to sit in with the psychologist when the patient returns and learn how to use desensitization techniques for managing anxiety. She would likely observe the psychologist model a guiding style, as opposed to the less effective, directive approach that is so common in busy primary care practices.

Let's return to the case of the woman in for a follow-up of her hypertension who was experiencing insomnia and anxiety since her daughter came to live with her. Imagine that this woman is presenting to the resident for help with her insomnia.

Resident	I have this woman who feels anxious and is not sleeping well. She is very upset about not being able to fall asleep.
Psychologist	It is key to ask her about what she is saying to herself—how she is making herself anxious. Likely, her mind has made the situation catastrophic. She may think she will always have trouble sleeping or that she can't live this way. These thoughts then trigger increased anxiety.
Resident	I can go back and talk to her about that.
Psychologist	I would point out the connection between her thoughts and anxiety. Then, I might ask her if she is open to a suggestion. If she is, I would suggest helping her see that the situation is not the end of the world.
Resident	How do I that?
Psychologist	You might talk with her about how we all have trouble sleeping from time to time. Ask her what it has been like the day after she sleeps poorly. Even though it is hard, has she been able to get through the day without losing her job or experiencing any major health problems? If so, would she be willing to simply go on with her days the best she can, go to bed at her usual time? She should get out of bed and read if she can't sleep, and then go back to bed once she is very sleepy. You could have her follow up with you to report on how this strategy worked. If she still is having trouble, I will be happy to see her.
Resident	Thanks

This resident is gaining confidence and learning an attitude about the value of assessing and treating the mental health of her patients by working as part of a comprehensive team.

The clinical skills needed to diagnose and treat mental health conditions in primary care might best be learned in the context of working as part of a collaborative team. No matter what system of education is used, the data are large and complex, requiring the primary care clinician to be a lifetime learner.

Mental Health Referral

The patient with insomnia and anxiety returns to see the resident several weeks after the intervention discussed above. She did not go to Alanon. Her daughter and her children continue to live with her. The patient and her daughter argue frequently. Her insomnia is no better.

Clinician	Let me see if I have it right so far. Your living situation has worsened. You are experiencing increased anxiety. Your insomnia is no better.
Patient	That's right. I'm not sure what to do about it.
Clinician	I have a suggestion. Would you like to hear it?
Patient	Sure.
Clinician	I think it would be a good idea to see a specialist who works with patients who have insomnia. I know a counselor who has helped a number of the patients in my practice. In fact, we work alongside each other. Have you ever gone for counseling help in the past?
Patient	No. I don't think it is that bad. Can we try something else first?
Clinician	What do you have in mind?
Patient	I think my sleep problems would resolve if my daughter would just move out.
Clinician	Do you think that is anything you have control over? For example, would you be willing to ask her to contribute financially, or find another place to live?
Patient	Not really.
Clinician	And, if she doesn't move out, you feel stuck and anxious?
Patient	Yes.
Clinician	Given that she may not move out and you are feeling anxious and tired, would you be interested learning ways of coping with a bad situation.
Patient	Tell me what you mean.
Clinician	We have discovered that people can learn a number of different techniques for helping themselves deal with anxiety and insomnia.

(continued)

> These are similar to the ones I discussed with you last time. Only,
> a counselor has the training to work closely with people and help
> them apply the techniques to their particular situation.
>
> **Patient**   Well, I would never make my daughter leave.
> **Clinician** I hear you. What do you think of my suggestion? We have a
>   counselor who works right here in our office.
> **Patient**   You mean I could see the counselor right here.
> **Clinician** Yes.
> **Patient**   That would be okay then.

This case highlights the key ingredients of an effective referral:

1. Guide the patient or family, rather than simply telling them they need to go see a mental health specialist [20]. Uncovering the patient or family motivation supports autonomy and is important since most mental health referrals fail [21]. Clinicians will have different thresholds for referral based on their training, experience, and the time they have available. Often, it is a good idea to have the patient or family return to discuss the situation further, before referring them, so they do not feel dismissed [22]. Referring to someone the clinician knows and trusts is likely to enhance collaboration. It is helpful to keep in mind that families functioning at a lower level frequently do not follow up on referrals to traditional therapy.
2. Ask about previous counseling experiences in order to avoid problems that may have occurred previously.
3. Use terms like consultation or counselor, instead of family therapist or psychologist, terms that some people think implies the family has a severe problem [22].
4. Use normalization to combat the stigma of a mental health referral: *Many families benefit from consulting with a specialist who has experience helping children open up and talk to their parents.*
5. Incorporate the family's language and belief systems into the discussion in order to get agreement to a specific plan [22].
6. Just like with any other behavioral change, it is important not to rush the process.

Key Points

1. The majority of patients with emotional or mental health problems are missed in primary care.
2. Sensitive specific psychosocial screens could identify many of those patients.
3. Primary care clinicians treat the majority of people who are treated for mental health conditions. They must develop skills for treating mental health conditions.

4. Good interviewing and relationship skills help many patients with emotional and mental health problems. These skills include engagement, partnership, and structuring.
5. The Collaborative Family Health Model addresses two important issues:

   (a) The high demand for mental health treatment in primary care
   (b) Ongoing need of primary care clinicians for education on mental health diagnosis and treatment

6. Effective referral to an outside mental health specialist takes a thoughtful approach.

References

1. Wang PS, Lane M, Ofsen M, Pincus HA, Wells KB, Kessler RC. The primary care of mental disorders in the United States. In: Manderscheid RW, Berry JT, editors. Mental health, United States, 2004. DHHS Pub. No. (SMA)-06-4195. Rockville, MD: Substance Abuse and Mental Health Services Administration; 2006.
2. Grandes G, Montoya I, Arietaleanizbeaskoa MS, Arce V, Sanchez A. The burden of mental disorders in primary care. Eur Psychiatry. 2011;26:428–35.
3. McDaniel SH, Fogarty CT. What primary care psychology has to offer the patient-centered medical home. Prof Psychol Res Pract. 2009;40:483–92.
4. Wissow L, Anthony B, Brown J, DosReis S, Gadomski A, Ginsberg G, et al. A common factors approach to improving the mental health capacity of pediatric primary care. Adm Policy Ment Health. 2008;35:305–18.
5. Deacon B, Lickel J, Abramowitz JS. Medical utilization across the anxiety disorders. J Anxiety Disord. 2008;22:344–50.
6. Sartorius N, Ustun TB, Lecrubier Y, Wittchen H-U. Depression co morbid with anxiety: results from the WHO study on psychological disorders in primary health care. Br J Psychiatry. 1996;168 Suppl 30:538–43.
7. Birmaher B, Rey JM. Treating child and adolescent depression. Philadelphia, PA: Lippincott Williams and Wilkins; 2009.
8. Jellinek MS, Murphy JM, Little M, Pagano ME, Comer DM, Kelleher KJ. Use of the pediatric symptom checklist (PSC) to screen for psychosocial problems in pediatric primary care: a national feasibility study. Arch Pediatr Adolesc Med. 1999;153:254–60.
9. Kroenke K, Spitzer RL, Williams JB. The PHQ – 9: validity of a brief depression severity measure. J Gen Intern Med. 2001;16:606–13.
10. Girón M, Majón-Arce P, Puerto-Barber J, Sánchez-Garcia E, Gómez-Beneyto M. Clinical interviewing skills and identification of emotional disorders in primary care. Am J Psychiatry. 1998;155:530–5.
11. Goldberg D, Steele JJ, Johnson A, Smith C. Ability of primary care physicians to make accurate ratings of psychiatric symptoms. Arch Gen Psychiatry. 1982;39:829–33.
12. Karver MS, Handelsman JB, Fields S, Bickman L. Meta-analysis of therapeutic relationship variables in youth and family therapy: the evidence for different relationship variables in the child and adolescent treatment outcome literature. Clin Psychol Rev. 2006;26:50–65.
13. Angold A, Costello EJ, Farmer EM, Burns BJ, Erkanli A. Impaired but undiagnosed. J Am Acad Child Adolesc Psychiatry. 1999;38:129–37.
14. Brown JD, Wissow LS, Riley AW. Physician and patient characteristics associated with discussion of psychosocial health during pediatric primary care visits. Clin Pediatr (Phila). 2007;46:812–20.

15. Hirschfeld RM, Williams JB, Spitzer RL, Calabrese JR, Flynn L, Keck PE Jr, et al. Development and validation of a screening instrument for bipolar spectrum disorder: the mood disorder questionnaire. Am J Psychiatry. 2000;157:1873–5.
16. Worthington JJ, Rauch SL. Approach to the patient with depression. In: Goroll AH, Mulley AG, editors. Primary care medicine: office evaluation of the adult patient. Philadelphia, PA: Lippincott Williams and Wilkins; 2009. Chapter 27.
17. Regaldo M, Halfen N. Primary care services promoting optimal child development from birth to age three years: a review of the literature. Arch Pediatr Adolesc Med. 2001;155:1311–22.
18. Olson AL, Kelleher KJ, Kemper KJ, Zuckerman BS, Hammond CS, Dietrich AJ. Primary care pediatrician's roles and perceived responsibilities in the identification and management of depression in children and adolescents. Ambul Pediatr. 2001;1:91–8.
19. Ries A. Pulmonary rehabilitation and COPD. Sem Resp Crit Care Med. 2005;26:133–41.
20. Rollnick S, Miller WR, Butler CC. Motivational interviewing in health care: helping patients change behavior. New York, NY: The Guilford Press; 2008.
21. Rushton J, Bruckmann D, Kelleher K. Primary care of children with psychosocial problems. Arch Pediatr Adolesc Med. 2002;156:592–8.
22. McDaniel SH, Campbell TC, Hepworth J, Lorenz A. Family-oriented primary care. 2nd ed. New York, NY: Springer; 2005.

Chapter 15
Body–Mind Integration

Role Play

Mastering of the following basic interviewing skills is necessary in order to be successful with the somatic fixation role plays: *maintain a slow pace and **listen**, obtain the **personal story**, join, **contract**, ask **open-ended inquiries**, obtain **theory of illness**, and give **affirmations***.

Role Play: A 55-year-old woman with depression and multiple physical complaints. She has difficulty walking because of weakness, although her neurological and muscular exams are normal. The patient attributes her weakness to an unspecified nutritional deficiency. The clinician believes the symptoms are emotionally based, exacerbated by a recent, second divorce.

Objective

Explain the patient's diagnosis using a strength-based approach.

Trainee	I would like to talk to you about your difficulty walking.
Patient	Okay.
Trainee	The weakness is interfering in your day to day life. You believe the main problem is a nutritional deficiency that we have not yet identified. I think that could be part of it. There is another important component: your emotions. I think your body is expressing feel-

(continued)

	ings that you are having difficulty saying in words. Our bodies do this all the time. We smile automatically and involuntarily when we are happy or have tears when we are sad.
Patient	The weakness is real, doctor.
Trainee	I know. I am just saying the stress you have been going through has contributed to your weakness.
Patient	If you say so.
Faculty	Would you like an option for dealing with the patient?
Trainee	Please.

Feedback

Faculty	I would suggest slowing down. It is true that she needs education about her diagnosis and how our bodies automatically express our feelings. However, her primary need at this point is acceptance and validation of her concerns. Yes, her body is telling her that it is now time to attend to her own needs. However, that has not been her framework for understanding her symptoms. She may not even perceive that she is experiencing stress. Her focus is somatic. I would suggest acknowledging her belief system and concerns with an empathic summary or two. Once she feels heard, ask her permission to share your perspective. She might be more receptive to a change in focus at that time.
Trainee	I think I have it. I'm ready to give it a shot.

Replay

Trainee	Could we take a minute to discuss your diagnosis?
Patient	Sure.
Trainee	Tell me how you see things.
Patient	I think the main problem is that I have a gluten sensitivity. I have been reading about it and I fit the picture exactly.
Trainee	Tell me more
Patient	I have read how our bodies can be allergic to gluten and that it can cause all kinds of problems with muscle and joint pain. That has

(continued)

> been my main problem. I started to go on a gluten-free diet, but
> I have not been strict about it, so I don't know yet if it will work.
>
> **Trainee** So, you have been researching your condition and discovered
> information about some folks having a gluten sensitivity. The
> symptoms fit your symptoms well, and you would like support as
> you start a gluten-free diet.
>
> **Patient** That's right.
>
> **Trainee** I think that could be part of it and I will work with you with on it.
> I also think there is something else, your emotions. You seem to
> me to be the type of person who has put her needs and feelings on
> the back burner. I believe that your body is saying "Enough—pay
> attention to me." It is like smiling automatically when somebody
> says something funny. You can't help yourself. Well, I believe the
> same thing is happening with your muscles now.
>
> **Patient** I still think the problem is the gluten.

Feedback

> **Faculty** Let's stop here. Nice job of listening and acknowledging her per-
> spective. Of course, patients will not always agree with our diag-
> nosis. We can still work collaboratively to help them feel better,
> while holding a different view of the problem. In fact, that is com-
> monly the situation with somatically fixated patients.

Obstacles to Teaching Body–Mind Integration

1. These families can be very challenging and foster a sense of helplessness in clinicians. This helplessness can be transmitted from mentor to student.
2. The patient and clinician have different belief systems. It can be difficult to integrate the biomedical and psychosocial.
3. It can be difficult for trainees to see and affirm the strengths in these patients and
   families.

Strategies

1. Empathize with the trainees' feelings. At the same time, help trainees not buy into
   a sense of helplessness with these families. The mentor can model a helpful approach
   and point out examples of families who have made progress, even if it is slow.

2. Use a biopsychosocial approach from the beginning. Don't focus solely on emotional factors. Solicit somatic symptoms. Ask about stress associated with those symptoms to move to the patient's emotional experiences [1]. Use examples to educate about mind–body connections: we smile automatically and involuntarily when happy; we feel butterflies in our stomachs when anxious; and experience headaches and insomnia when stressed [2].
3. Encourage trainees to find things they like or respect about the patient early on in their relationship. Give the trainee-specific examples of affirming statements they can make.

Body–Mind Integration

> Joseph is an 11-year-old obese child who has a follow up appointment for high blood pressure, noted on a routine checkup. The family changed their diet after the last visit. Joseph lost weight. He increased his activity level. Today, his blood pressure is in the normal range. However, Joseph is experiencing recurrent chest pain and appears anxious. Joseph's theory of illness, obtained using the third-person technique, involves a heart problem. The mother fills in the details. At the last visit, the clinician thought he heard something wrong with his heart. Since that time Joseph has worried. His worry and his chest pain are resolvable with clear information.

Good health care requires the integration of both the physical and emotional/social dimensions of illness. Patients commonly experience anxiety about their physical illnesses, present with the somatic manifestations of depression and anxiety, have psychosomatic conditions, or focus exclusively on the somatic aspects of complex, chronic illnesses [1]. Sometimes, patients are aware and readily accept the connection between the mind and body, like the family in the above case. Other times, they focus on the physical dimension despite little or no evidence that the physical is playing a significant role. These patients are among the most challenging a primary care clinician cares for in the course of his or her day.

Somatically fixated patients present with an exclusive focus on physical symptoms in the face of very difficult life circumstances, discounting the emotional dimension [1]. Severe somatization is associated with a history of neglect or abuse, and a family history of somatization as a way of coping [3, 4]. Some patients may be diagnosed with a psychiatric disorder, one of the somatoform disorders, such as psychogenic pain disorder.

Although patients who focus on the somatic dimensions of a condition are challenging, a thoughtful interviewing approach, using a biopsychosocial model, can help the clinician stay out of a struggle with patients who emphasize the physical dimension.

Interviewing Strategies

The first task, as with all patients, is creating emotional safety. The clinician must be aware and resolve any underlying frustration or annoyance so that he or she can be fully present to the patient. One way to accomplish this is through listening to the patient's personal story [5]. As the clinician understands the patient's suffering, the clinician is likely to experience empathy. Empathic summaries are important tools in helping the patient feel understood. A summary can also be used to guide the interview when the patient is stuck on an excessively long description of the physical symptoms [1].

Patient	My belly has been troubling me on and off for some time now.
Clinician	Let me see if I have heard you accurately. You have had trouble with your bowels for a long time. You have also experienced abdominal pain off and on and it has been quite distressing... Nothing we have tried has given you relief. Is that right? (*patient nods*) Let me now move to another area for a bit and ask you....

Another component of establishing emotional safety is agreeing to a clear contract: *Lots of medical problems can cause the type of problems you are experiencing—intestinal inflammation, food intolerances, as well as stresses people face in their day-to-day life. I am going to be asking you questions about all those areas.* Both elements of the patient's functioning are given priority, not treated as unrelated processes. The biomedical is not worked up, and then the psychosocial causes investigated if no biomedical answer uncovered. This leads to patient resistance: *You think it is all in my head.*

In addition to the above core interviewing strategies, McDaniel et al. list a number of principles that help the clinician stay out of a struggle with his or her patient. Among them, are the following [1].

Negotiate a Mutually Acceptable Diagnosis

The clinician elicits the meaning of the symptom to the patient and family, and works from that understanding to a mutually acceptable diagnosis that incorporates biomedical and psychosocial aspects [1, 5]. The following summary includes the patient's perspective:

Clinician	Let's talk about the cause of your recurrent abdominal pain. Likely, several elements contribute. I do think your idea of the foods you eat adversely affecting you is part of it. I also think you have a tendency to be stoic and keep a "stiff upper lip," which might contribute. What do you think of that possibility? [2]
Patient	That is possible.

Invite the Family to Participate Early in Treatment

The family members present at a family conference can facilitate moving the patient from a purely biomedical to a biopsychosocial focus. The meaning of the symptom as it relates to family interactions becomes clear via direct or circular questioning.

Clinician	Have you noticed any pattern to your wife's abdominal pain.
Husband	It seems to me that any type of stress can bring it on. It could be a worry about the finances or the children, or when she and I are not getting along particularly well. Neither one of us likes conflict.

Affirm the Patient and Family's Strengths

Patients with a history of neglect or abuse are very sensitive to any judgment on the part of the clinician. Building on their strengths leads to collaboration. Watson recommends the patient's psychological defense be framed positively, as in the following statement [2, 6].

Clinician	You seem to me to be the type of person who puts other people's needs first. You let your own needs take a back seat. A part of you, your body, is screaming for acknowledgement, for you to pay attention.
Patient	I have always been that way.

Avoid Psychosocial Fixation

Balance the biomedical and psychosocial. Somatically fixated patients get physical illnesses, too. They also undergo unnecessary tests. The astute clinician avoids missing physical illnesses by paying attention to red flags, such as weight loss or fever. The clinician avoids unnecessary tests by making the diagnosis of a functional condition, when appropriate, and stopping the workup.

Judge Progress by Monitoring Changes in Functioning

Help the patient gradually adopt a more healthful lifestyle. Improved functioning, not cure, is an attainable goal. The focus should not stay on the symptoms, but on what activities a patient can do to be more active and feel better [5].

Key Points

1. Avoid being frustrated with these patients by getting to know their suffering through their personal story.
2. Contract to evaluate both psychological and physical factors.
3. Solicit the patient's symptoms. Gain access to their emotional experience by inquiring into the stress associated with the physical symptoms.
4. Understand the patient's and family's theory of illness and symbolic meaning.
5. Include patient's theory of illness in formulation of problem.
6. Affirm strengths of patient and family.
7. Focus on improving function, not cure.

References

1. McDaniel SH, Campbell TL, Hepworth J, Lorenz A. Family-oriented primary care. 2nd ed. New York, NY: Springer; 2005.
2. Watson W. Bridging the mind-body split towards an integrated framework for thinking about somatoform symptoms. Fam Psychol. 2007;23(1):30–3.
3. Katon W. Somatization in primary care. J Fam Pract. 1985;21:257–8.
4. Livingston R, Witt A, Smith GR. Families who somatize. J Dev Behav Pediatr. 1995;16:42–6.
5. Platt FW, Gordon GH. Field guide to the difficult patient interview. 2nd ed. Philadelphia, PA: Lippincott, Williams and Wilkins; 2004.
6. Watson W. From the president: somatoform disorders and the family: clinical impressions-part 1. Fam Psychol. 2007;23(1):42–4.

Chapter 16
Suicide Assessment

Role Play

The following prerequisite interviewing skills need to be mastered before role-playing suicidal assessments: maintain a slow pace, elicit feelings, *empathic summary, feeling response, self-awareness*, clarify vague answers, *open-ended inquiry, validity tools* for increasing accuracy, and *transitional statements*.

Role Play #1:   A 60 yr. old woman with worsening depression is on an antidepressant. She has severe arthritis, and quit work one year ago. She lives on her own.

Objectives

1. Set the platform to inquire about suicidal thinking and behavior.
2. Use a behavioral incident to carefully carve out current suicidal thinking and behavior.

Trainee	Mrs. Jones, you say your depression is worse and the medicine doesn't seem to help. Tell me about it.
Patient	I can't get myself going in the morning. My sleep is bad.
Trainee	It sounds tough. Say more about it.
Patient	I get four to five hours of sleep a night. I feel lousy when I wake up and find it hard to get myself activated.
Trainee	Hard to get activated?
Patient	Yes. I have always been someone who was active. I worked for 30 years, and hardly missed a day. I feel lost.

(continued)

Trainee	How do you mean "lost"?
Patient	I don't know. I used to have a purpose with my work. Now, I feel disorganized. I wished I had a focus.
Trainee	It sounds difficult
Patient	It is.
Trainee	So, you feel lost and have no focus. When you are feeling at your worst, do you have times when you just wish your life was over?
Patient	I do wish that at times.
Trainee	Have you had thoughts of killing yourself?
Patient	Sometimes
Trainee	Do the thoughts come and go or there all the time?
Patient	I have them every day.
Trainee	Have you made a plan to kill yourself?
Patient	No.
Trainee	Ok, I think we are finished.

Feedback

Faculty	Affirmations?
Trainee #2	You clarified whether she was having suicidal thinking, not just passive thoughts. You had a good pace and appeared calm.
Faculty	Yes, in addition you had a nice empathic statement when she mentioned her sleep problem. You set the platform nicely by asking what she was experiencing and not rushing through it. And you summarized well. Very nice. I have one option. I would explore her current suicidal thinking more fully. These four questions, taken directly from Managing Suicide Risk in Primary Care, will help you more fully carve this region. (1) Have you thought about how you might kill yourself? (2) When you think about suicide, do the thoughts come and go, or are they so intense you can't think about anything else? (3) Have you practiced in any way, or have you done anything to prepare for your death? (4) Do you have access to (method)? (See Table 16.1.) I wrote them down on a card. Let's run through it one more time. You can refer to this card during the interview, if you want.
Trainee	Okay. I'm ready to go again.

Table 16.1 Sequencing risk assessment questions for BHCs

1. *Suicide screening*
   - Many times when people feel [describe symptoms or complaints] they also think about death or have thoughts about suicide. Do you ever wish you were dead or think about killing yourself?
   - Do things ever get so bad you think about ending your life or suicide?
2. *Differentiate suicidal ideation from nonsuicidal morbid ideation*
   - Tell me a little bit about what, specifically, you have been thinking.
   - What is it exactly that goes through your mind?
   - When you think about dying, is it because you have caused it to happen?
3. *Assess for past suicidal behaviors*
   - Have you ever had thoughts like this before?
   - Have you ever intentionally injured yourself in any way before?
   - Have you ever tried to kill yourself before?
   - So you've never cut yourself, burned yourself, held a gun to your head, taken more pills than you should, or tried to kill yourself in any other way?
4. *If positive history of suicidal behaviors, assess multiple attempt status*
   - How many times have you tried to kill yourself?
   - Let's talk about the first time...
     (a) When did this occur?
     (b) What did you do?
     (c) Where were you when you did this?
     (d) Did you hope you would die, or did you hope something else would happen?
     (e) Afterward, were you glad to be alive or disappointed you weren't dead?
   - Let's talk a little bit about the worst time you attempted suicide; the time you were most suicidal and tried to kill yourself...
   [Repeat (a) through (e) above]
5. *Assess current suicidal episode*
   - Let's talk about what's going on right now. You said you've been thinking about [content].
   - Have you thought about how you might kill yourself?
   - When you think about suicide, do the thoughts come and go, or are they so intense you can't think about anything else?
   - Have you practiced [method] in any way, or have you done anything to prepare for your death?
   - Do you have access to [method]?
6. *Screen for protective factors*
   - With all that's been going on, what is keeping you alive right now?
   - What prevents you from killing yourself?

Copied with permission from **Managing Suicide Risk in Primary Care (2011) by Byran and Rudd**

Replay

Trainee	Tell me how you think your medicine for depression is working.
Patient	It does not seem to be working. I can't get myself going in the morning.
Trainee	Tell me more about it.
Patient	I have always been an active person. I worked for 30 years, and hardly missed a day. I feel lost.
Trainee	How do you mean "lost"?
Patient	I don't know. I used to have a purpose with my work. Now, I feel disorganized. I wished I had a focus.
Trainee	It sounds difficult
Patient	It is.
Trainee	When you are feeling real bad do you have thoughts of ending your life, of suicide?
Patient	Sometimes.
Trainee	Would it be okay if I ask a few questions about those thoughts?
Patient	Go ahead.
Trainee	Have you thought about how you might kill yourself?
Patient	I have thought of taking all my pills. I haven't considered anything else.
Trainee	When you think about suicide, do the thoughts come and go, or are they so intense you can't think about anything else?
Patient	They come and go. I rarely think about it.
Trainee	Have you practiced in any way, or have you done anything to prepare for your death? For example, have you picked up the pill bottle with thoughts of taking an overdose?
Patient	No, I would never do it. I don't want to leave my grandchildren.
Trainee	Do you have easy access to pills.
Patient	They are right there in my medicine cabinet.

Feedback

Faculty	Good job. You got a clearer picture of her current suicidal thinking.

Role Play #2:   Melissa is a 14-year-old girl in your office after her mother discovered her diary detailing cutting behavior. Melissa is upset. Both her parents are present. She has no history of suicidal ideation or behavior in the past. She has been depressed for a year and has been cutting herself.

Objectives

1. Ask adolescent about suicidal thoughts.
2. Check out family perspective.

Trainee	I am Dr. Black.
Parents	Hi. We are Bob and Stacy Shaw. This is Melissa.
Trainee	Before we get started talking about the reason for today's visit, I am going to ask you to tell me a little about yourselves. I like to get to know people as people before discussing their medical concerns. Is that okay with you?
Everyone	Yes.
Trainee	Melissa, let's start with you. Tell me about yourself.
Patient	What do you mean?
Trainee	Who are the important people in your life? What do you like to do? How is school, family? Whatever you think it would be important for me to know.
Patient	I'm a sophomore in school. I am in the band. Most of my friends are members of the band. I play the clarinet.
Trainee	How long have you played the clarinet?
Patient	Two years.
Trainee	I imagine you like it?
Patient	I do like it a lot.
Trainee	So, you are a sophomore in high school. You are in the band along with your friends. Tell me more.
Patient	I have 2 brothers. My older brother goes to my high school. We get along okay.
Trainee	Good. Let me switch to you, Mrs. Shaw. Tell me about yourself.
Mother	I am a paralegal. I work in a lawyer's office part time. We have three children. Melissa is the middle child. I am very concerned about her right now.
Trainee	We will get to that in 1 minute. Would you say more about yourself?
Mother	I think her father and I have both had stresses between work and his family. Bob's father died a year ago. He was very close to Melissa. In addition, I have had some medical problems and had to go through some testing, recently.

(continued)

Trainee	Say more about yourself.
Mother	I am close to my children. They are my number one priority. However, I have not been as available to the children since I became ill.
Trainee	So, you have been facing a lot of change and stress as a family.
Father	Yes, my mother now lives by herself. I have been busy helping her and have not been around as much as I used to be.
Trainee	Not around as much as you used to be?
Father	My mother can be demanding. I want to help as much as I can, but I have only so much time.
Trainee	It does sound like it has been a lot to deal with.
Mother	It has been a challenge. Our biggest concern is Melissa.
Trainee	Tell me more about your concerns. I do know a little bit from your call to me yesterday, Mrs. Shaw.
Mother	As I was telling you yesterday, I discovered that Melissa and a friend have been cutting on themselves. I am real worried about her.
Trainee	Melissa, is there anything else that you want to make sure we discuss during today's visit
Patient	No.
Trainee	I am going to shift gears now… I would like to talk to you all about today's visit. Melissa, I plan to talk with you alone for part of the visit. Afterwards, I would like to talk with you and your parents together. I will keep everything private. I do this so you can feel free to talk with me. There is one exception. If you tell me anything that makes me concerned about your safety, or the safety of someone else, I would talk with your parents about it. Is that plan okay with you?
Melissa	Yes.

Parents also agree and then leave the room.

Trainee	Tell me your perspective on the situation. Do you know your mother called and gave me a brief overview yesterday?
Patient	Yes. She got all upset when she found out I have been cutting.
Trainee	Before you tell me about the cutting, I would first like to ask you some questions that will help me better understand the bigger picture.
Patient	Okay.

(continued)

Trainee	How has your overall mood been in the last two weeks?
Patient	I've been down.
Trainee	What do you mean?
Patient	I have not felt like myself. I don't feel like doing anything. I have to force myself to do my homework, and it takes me forever.
Trainee	Sounds difficult. Say more about that.
Patient	I don't know what is going on. Sometimes I feel really bad.
Trainee	Really bad?
Patient	It is hard to explain.
Trainee	I imagine it is confusing to feel bad and not know why.
Patient	It has been hard.
Trainee	When people feel really bad they often have thoughts of killing themselves. Is that true for you?
Patient	Not really.
Trainee	What thoughts have you had?
Patient	I've wondered what it would be like to die.
Trainee	When you think of dying is it because you caused it to happen.
Patient	No, I never thought that.

The trainee goes on to obtain details about Melissa's depression, the cutting, and her view of family relationships. The parents are then invited back into the office.

Trainee	Mr. and Mrs. Shaw, I would like to hear your perspective.
Mother	I am very concerned. I found her writing about cutting herself. She and her best friend have been doing this for quite a while. We took away all sharp objects. We are watching her constantly. I don't know when I will be able to trust her again.
Father	I am very concerned. She has been spending too much time in her room. I know teenagers do that, but I think she needs to be more involved with the family. We have always done things together. We are a close family.
Patient	Okay, I'll spend more time with you.
Mother	There is the note in her diary. I think it was a suicidal note.
Patient	Mom, it is not a suicidal note.
Mother	What is it?
Patient	I just have not been myself. I don't know what is wrong.
Trainee	Let me jump in here. Melissa, you have a clinical depression. The cutting has been your attempt to cope with very painful feelings. You were very close to your grandpa and he died last year. Your mom has

(continued)

been dealing with a serious medical problem and you have been worried about her. Adding to your losses, you have felt ostracized by some of the kids at school. This has all contributed to your depression. The depression is treatable.

Mother I knew she was not herself. The cutting has really upset me. We are going to have to watch her constantly.

Trainee Let's talk about safety.

Feedback

Faculty Okay, great job, let's stop. (*to trainee*) What did you like about your interview?

Trainee I thought I had a good connection with the patient and family. I tried to be thorough. I explained what I was doing all along.

Faculty Other affirmations?

Mother I thought you listened carefully to my concerns. You took everybody's view into account.

Trainee #2 You used normalization to ask about suicide. You said that people often have thoughts of suicide when they feel real bad.

Trainee #3 You did a great job staying calm, even though the parents were upset about the cutting.

Faculty You did a careful assessment. You addressed privacy issues. You got a personal story. I think that was a good way to begin since you didn't know the family. You set the platform before asking about suicide. You had a good structure for the interview. I like the way you brought the parents in to get their perspective. It is important to get collateral data to make sure you are not missing anything. Also, you saw they want to be supportive. That is crucial data.

Trainee Thanks.

Faculty Does anybody have options?

Group (*no response*)

Faculty I have one. I noticed that your pace became a little fast at times. Did you notice that?

Trainee Yes, I think you are right.

Faculty Good awareness. It is very easy to hurry when there is so much crucial data to obtain. It is important to go slowly when doing a suicide assessment, so the patient feels safe to talk. If you stay aware, you can take a breath, slow yourself down and be fully present.

Trainee Thanks. I will keep that in mind.

Role Play #3:   Melissa, age 14, and her family. Continue where Role Play #2 concluded.

Objectives

1. Establish a clear contract to perform means restriction counseling
2. Use an empathic summary if family has difficulty with this issue

Trainee	I would like to talk to you about one more topic. Melissa has depression and we know that is a risk factor for suicide. We all want to help her feel better and stop suffering. In order to do that, it is important that she stay safe and alive. Even though Melissa has stated she is not suicidal, depression can feel unbearable at times and lead to suicidal thoughts. Therefore, I would like to talk with you about making the environment safe. You know, firearms, knifes, pills,... Is that okay with you?
Mother	Sure
Father	Of course I want my daughter to be safe. But, I have always had a gun. I am a hunter and gun collector.
Trainee	You have always owned a gun. I imagine the thought of removing firearms sounds like a huge step. Of course, you want to keep your daughter safe.
Father	Yes.
Trainee	Well, let's look at our options. We are not talking about a permanent situation.
Father	Okay. How long are we talking about?
Trainee	I would recommend removing firearms out of the house for minimum of six months after the depression has resolved.
Father	I will take care of that today.
Trainee	I would like to write our safety plan down so we are all on the same page.

Feedback

Faculty	Let's stop. Wonderful job. You obtained a clear contract. You did not debate with the father. Instead you used an empathic summary. This helped you maintain a partnership with him based on the common goal of alleviating Melissa's suffering. Finally, you were open to collaborating with the father and informed him this was a temporary approach. (See section on Means Restriction Counseling.)

Obstacles to Teaching Suicide Assessment

1. Interviewer has a hidden belief (e.g., suicide is a sign of weakness) that interferes with a nonjudgmental attitude.
2. Fear of dealing with intense dysphoria.
3. There is limited time for role plays. Learning how to perform a good suicidal assessment takes repetition and time.
4. Lack of knowledge.

Strategies

1. Use group process to discuss clinician's attitudes and thinking when assessing suicide.
2. Empathize with the learner. Explore what underlies the clinician's fear, and normalize reactions. Faculty member can demonstrate techniques for dealing with intense affect.
3. Set aside enough time. It is an essential skill for all clinicians!
4. Teach a sequential and hierarchical method that is both efficient and readily learnable.

Suicide Assessment in Primary Care

Forty-five percent of people who die by suicide contact a primary care clinician in the month before their deaths [1]. An opportunity exists for primary care clinicians to identify high-risk individuals and intervene to prevent suicides [2, 3]. It is important for a primary care clinician to have a systematic, organized approach. Most mistakes in suicide assessment are made as a result of errors of omission, distortion, and false assumptions, rather than as a result of bad decisions with a complete database [4]. The patient's risk factors and the patient's unique suicidal thinking and plans comprise the essential elements of a complete database [5]. The focus in this chapter is on practical interviewing strategies that a primary care clinician or a behavioral health consultant working in primary care can utilize to uncover a patient's unique suicidal thinking and plans. The first strategy is staying self-aware.

Interfering Cognitions

Establishing an atmosphere that supports emotional contact and safety to talk can be extraordinarily difficult with a patient who feels shame, harboring a suicidal secret. Many patients have strong negative beliefs about their own suicidal thinking. Some believe suicidal thoughts represent a character weakness or signify that they are crazy; others see suicidality as a sinful or taboo subject; and many believe nobody can help them, so they see no purpose for sharing their secret [4].

Physicians also hold any number of beliefs and attitudes that can create a strong emotional reaction and interfere with a good suicidal assessment. Physicians, like patients, may consider suicide as a sign of weaknesses, craziness, or sin; they may consider suicide a taboo subject, or the situation to be hopeless. A physician holding onto any of those beliefs will convey judgment or disapproval to the patient. A patient attuned to the nonverbal signals of the clinician, such as a disapproving face, fast pace, or change in the tone of voice, may assume disapproval and then remain alone with his or her secret [4].

A second group of beliefs and attitudes, just as incapacitating as the first group, almost always remain covert. A physician who uncovers suicidal thinking or behavior will need to spend extra time and energy in order to properly evaluate and triage that patient [4]. In addition, appropriate mental health referrals can be difficult to access. A busy clinician might hope that a patient is not suicidal, so he or she would not be required to spend the extra time evaluating the patient. Although an understandable desire, it is damaging to convey this wish to a patient who is already ambivalent about sharing a suicidal secret. Shea lists another clinician attitude that interferes with a competent suicide assessment: clinicians want to avoid anxiety. No clinician wants to worry about a patient when he or she finishes the workday and goes home to family, worry that can be expected by the clinician who has triaged a suicidal patient earlier that day [4]. Instead of fleeing from this anxiety, the clinician must face it directly by considering and answering two questions [4]:

• What am I feeling right now?
• Is there any part of me that doesn't want to hear the truth right now?

A clinician establishes an atmosphere of safety by first doing a careful self-examination and resolving any internal biases. The clinician must then help diminish the shame that many patients experience with suicidal thinking. This shame results from deeply held beliefs about suicidality, noted above. A direct confrontation of these beliefs usually leads to a defensive reaction and poor engagement. The clinician needs a softer approach. Shea suggests two specific strategies for addressing this shame and secrecy: setting the platform and use of validity techniques [4].

Setting the Platform

The more we understand our patients' suffering, the more engaged we can be with our patients. By talking about their suffering, patients will be more likely to share their suicidal state as they seek relief from a painful depression or a state of "crises, anger, anxiety, and hopelessness" [4]. The interviewer enters into the patient's experience of pain and uses that as a gateway to ask about suicidality. Asking about suicidality in that context feels natural and not like the question has been "popped" [4]. Two conclusions result from this understanding of suicidal assessment:

1. Establishing a strong engagement in order to obtain a full database takes on added importance when performing a suicide assessment. A hurried pace is likely to disengage the patient; it is important for a clinician to monitor his or her pace.
2. Since the patient's nonverbal signs (e.g., fidgetiness, avoidance of eye contact) communicate information of which he or she may be unaware, it is particularly important for the clinician to stay fully present and attuned to the patient.

A primary care clinician must decide who to assess for suicidal thoughts and behaviors. Since suicide is the leading cause of death in 15–19-year-olds, the American Academy of Child and Adolescent Psychiatry recommends screening this group for current and past suicidal ideation/behavior, substance abuse, and depression [6]. The U.S. Preventive Services Task Force does not encourage or discourage screening in adults because of insufficient evidence to make a recommendation [3]. The adult clinician might respond to this USPSTF position in one of several ways:

1. Use a questionnaire, such as the PHQ-9 to screen all patients for depression and suicide. The sensitivity and specificity of this instrument are adequate [7].
2. Ask about suicidality in select patients, such as those with depression, other mental health disorders, or physical conditions complicated by disability. The advantage of this approach is that it can be done without placing a burden on the practice to assess, track, and treat a large number of identified patients. A critical disadvantage is that it misses the vast majority of patients and the opportunity to treat those patients—potentially decreasing morbidity and mortality [8].

Once the patient is fully engaged with the interviewer and in touch with the psychic pain of the suicidal state, the clinician inquires about suicidal ideation [4]. If a patient appears anxious, the clinician might start off with a mildly ambiguous question, as a gentle way to bring up the topic of suicide [4]. *Are there ever times when you wish your life were over?*

The clinician would follow this question with a specific inquiry into thoughts of killing oneself.

Normalization

In the following example with an adolescent, depression is used as the gateway to a suicidal inquiry. **Normalization** is used to increase the likelihood of accurate reporting by the patient.

Patient	My friends get on my nerves. Most of the time, I just hang out in my room.
Clinician	What's that like?
Patient	I feel really bad. I'm all alone.
Clinician	Tell me about being alone.
Patient	It feels like no one cares about me (*looks sad*). I don't have anyone to talk to besides my dog.
Clinician	(slows pace, softens voice) You feel alone. Tell me more about that.
Patient	I don't know. I cry sometimes. I feel so all alone. Even my best friend Shelly has abandoned me. She doesn't call me anymore.
Clinician	It sounds difficult. Lots of folks who feel alone and down in the dumps have thoughts of wishing their life was over. Is that true for you? (*normalization*)
Patient	Sometimes.
Clinician	Have you thought of ending it all, of killing yourself?
Comment	*The clinician asks directly about killing oneself or being suicidal—not just hurting oneself. This area is too important to have miscommunication about what the patient means [9].*

Database

A positive response to a suicidal inquiry leads to a full suicidal assessment. Wishing one were dead without specific suicidal thinking (*It would be okay if I didn't wake up in the morning*) is not considered a positive screen. Since these patients have a lower suicidal risk, a different clinical response is required, such as treating the underlying condition and monitoring their morbid ideation regarding death [10].

The database in a suicide assessment may be large. An organized, systematic interview is required to gather all the data needed to make a sound diagnosis and treatment plan. "Winging it" is a common human response when facing a potentially large database [11]. "Winging it" results in errors of omission. Splitting the data into a sequence of smaller regions allows the clinician to more easily recall the information needed for each region [11].

Several methods for sequencing and organizing the patient's unique suicidal experience have widespread clinical acceptance [10, 11]. The CASE (Chronological Assessment of Suicidal Events) method sequences the data into four separate time regions; each region is associated with specific techniques to enhance accuracy [11]. The CASE method has been successfully taught to mental health professionals, as well as primary care clinicians via macrotraining [11]. Macrotraining utilizes repetitive role plays to achieve overlearning the material [11].

Bryan and Rudd describe a second empirically based sequencing method. The data collected are prioritized according to its predictive value for suicidal behavior. This is time efficient, and important, given the time limits inherent in primary care [10]. Evidence has supported these questions, among hundreds that could be asked about risk factors, as having the greatest risk of suicide. Primary care clinicians and behavioral health consultants working in primary care do not have time to ask hundreds of questions. However, they do have time to build the history together, weaving in open-ended questions, such as: *Tell me about the first time you tried to kill yourself* [10]. Questions are sequenced so that patient anxiety is decreased and, consequently, accuracy is increased. The clinician begins with less emotionally intense questions, and then moves to repetitive, highly specific questions as the patient becomes comfortable discussing suicide [4].

Once a clinician has determined that the patient needs a suicide assessment, he or she must evaluate risk factors. Risk factors include predisposition to suicidal behavior (e.g., history of psychiatric diagnosis, history of abuse), identifiable precipitant or stressors, symptomatic presentation (e.g., current mood symptoms), presence of hopelessness, previous suicidal behavior, impulsivity, self-control (e.g., substance abuse), access to lethal means, protective factors, and **the nature of the suicidal thinking** [12]. As previously noted, this chapter focuses on asking about the actual suicidal thoughts and behaviors of the patient.

A synopsis of Bryan and Rudd's sequencing structure for assessing suicidal thoughts and behaviors from *Managing Suicidal Risk in Primary Care* follows. It was the structure used for the role-play scenarios at the beginning of the chapter.

Assess for Past Suicidal Behaviors

Past suicidal behavior is "the single most significant and robust predictor of future suicide attempts and death by suicide across the entire life span" [10]. The likelihood of accuracy in this area is enhanced by gradually increasing the intensity of questions:

Have you ever had thoughts of suicide like this before?
Have you ever tried to kill yourself before?

If the second question is answered negatively, a third question follows:

So, you've never cut yourself, burned yourself, held a gun to your head, taken more pills than you should, or tried to kill yourself in any other way? [10]

Denial of the specific technique potentially increases accuracy. For example, a patient, who has held a gun to his head, might say he has not tried to kill himself, since he didn't pull the trigger, and then answer the denial of the specific question honestly.

Screen for Multiple Attempts and Assess Attempt History

A patient with a history of past suicidal behavior is asked about the first episode and the most serious episode (Table 16.1). The worst-point suicide attempt is more closely associated with future suicidal behavior than the current crises in chronic attempters [13]. This past information reveals the patient's behavioral pattern and intent over time, and contributes to a good management plan for the current episode [10].

Assess the Current Suicidal Episode

Since most patients will not report a history of prior suicidal behavior, the clinician can move directly to current suicidal thinking. The clinician might move to this area with a transition statement: *Earlier you were telling me about your thoughts of ending your life. Tell me more.*

The clinician wants to create a "verbal videotape" of the patient's suicidal thinking and behavior [11]. He or she tracks carefully with the patient, filling in any missing information with the following focused questions:

Have you thought about how you might kill yourself?
When you think about suicide, do your thoughts come and go, or are they so intense you can't think about anything else?
Have you practiced [method] in any way or have you done anything to prepare for your death?
Do you have access to [method]?

[10, p. 78]

If a patient is hesitant to talk, the clinician can simply ask the patient what he or she thinks would happen if he or she were to disclose fully. In that way, any block to openness is made overt and can be discussed [10]. If the patient does not answer questions directly, or even if the patient does, collateral information from family, friends, professionals, and others can be invaluable. It is crucial in adolescent evaluations [14].

Screen for Protective Factors

The patient's reasons for living are supported with a back-and-forth conversation, not simply listed. Protective factors do not eliminate risk factors, but are part of the total picture and often provide clues for developing interventions and management strategies [10].

Means Restricting Counseling

Since most patients in primary care are not directly admitted to the hospital, a crises response plan (CRP) is needed. This is a written plan developed collaboratively with the patient as an aid to follow during a period of crisis [10]. Part of working with patients, families, and other support systems during a crisis entails limiting access to firearms and other means of suicide. Means restriction counseling is supported by expert opinion as an important risk management strategy [15]. Bryan et al. recently published a protocol they have used successfully for means restriction counseling with suicidal patients [15]. The protocol outlines an approach developed to avoid an adversarial relationship—a potential consequence of recommending removal of firearms or other means of suicide, such as pills, from the environment. The interviewing steps include:

1. Join with the patient. Restricting means is very difficult for some patients. Take an empathic stance and do not argue. Alleviating suffering is a common goal around which the patient and clinician can join without arguing [15].
2. Present a menu of options. For example, if a patient is unwilling to remove a gun from the home, the following options can be suggested: "Dismantle firearm and give critical piece to significant other; store firearm in tamper-proof safe secured by a significant other; completely remove ammunition" [15]. Hiding the firearm would not be offered as an option since that is not safe. All firearms are identified and handled similarly.
3. Use a means receipt to ensure that the plan has been implemented. The receipt is a written agreement between the patient and clinician. It is signed by a significant other and returned. It includes the specifics of what is being restricted, how it is being restricted, and the specific conditions under which the means will be returned. The temporary time frame can instill hope for the patient and reduce resistance [15].

Note

The primary care clinician must also be knowledgeable about treatment options in order to discuss them with the patient. This holds whether the patient has been referred to specialty care, or the clinician provides primary treatment of an underlying mental condition, such as depression. McDaniel et al. recommend that "All patients with active suicidal thoughts should be referred to a mental health professional, and those with plans need urgent evaluation. Those with the means and intent to commit suicide usually need immediate hospitalization." [16, p. 352].

One common area of misinformation regarding treatment relates to the Food and Drug Administration's 2004 black box warning on selective serotonin reuptake inhibitor (SSRI) antidepressant use in patients 24 years and younger. Misunderstanding of the warning by both clinicians and patients may have had the unintended consequences of reducing prescriptions of SSRIs, without stimulating a compensatory increase in other forms of treatment of depression (e.g., Cognitive Behavioral Therapy), for children, adolescents, and young adults [17, 18]. This change in clinical practice has been temporally associated with an increase in completed suicides in children and adolescents [18]. (For a full discussion, see Rudd et al. [17] and Bryan and Rudd [10].)

Key Points

1. Learning to screen and assess suicidal ideation/behavior well takes practice and repetition.
2. A sequential and hierarchal assessment approach provides essential information efficiently. This is important given the time constraints in primary care.
3. Sequencing the order of questioning can minimize patient anxiety and lead to more accurate self-report.
4. A large database is much easier to learn when organized into distinct, smaller regions.
5. Most suicidal assessment errors are made from omission, distortion, and false assumptions—not bad clinical decisions, made with a full and accurate database.
6. Techniques to increase accuracy are essential when asking about suicidal ideation because of the shame some patients experience.
7. Vague answers need to be clarified.
8. Repetitively inquiring into the key aspects of a patient's thinking decreases the likelihood that he or she will omit important data.
9. A past history of suicidal behavior is the most significant predictor of future suicidal attempts and death.
10. It is important for clinicians to take a collaborative approach; attempts to talk the patient out of suicidal thinking lead to resistance. Relief of suffering is a common goal.
11. Talk to third parties to assess any discrepancies.
12. Family involvement is crucial in adolescent evaluations.
13. Means restriction counseling is based on expert opinion.

References

1. Luoma JB, Martin CE, Pearson JL. Contact with mental health and primary care providers before suicide: a review of the evidence. Am J Psychiatry. 2002;159:909–16.
2. Shulberg HC, Hyg MS, Bruce ML, Lee PW, Williams JW, Dretrich AJ. Preventing suicide in primary care patients: the primary care physician's role. Gen Hosp Psychiatry. 2006;26:337–45.

3. U.S. Preventive Services Task Force. Screening to identify primary care patients who are at risk for suicide: recommendations from the U.S. preventive services task force. Ann Intern Med. 2004;140:820–35.

4. Shea SC. The practical art of suicide assessment: a guide for mental health professionals and substance abuse counselors. Hoboken, NJ: Wiley; 2002.

5. Shea SC. The delicate art of eliciting suicidal ideation. Psychiatr Ann. 2004;34:385–400.

6. American Academy of Child and Adolescent Psychiatry. Practice parameters for the assessment and treatment of children and adolescents with suicide behavior. J Am Acad Child Adolesc Psychiatry. 2001;40(suppl):24s–51s.

7. Kroenke K, Spitzer RL, Williams JB. The PHQ-9: validity of a brief depression severity measure. J Gen Intern Med. 2001;16:606–16.

8. Bryan CJ, Corso K, Rudd MD, Cordero L. Improving identification of suicidal patients in primary care through routine screening. Prim Care Community Psychiatr. 2008;13:143–7.

9. Binder J. Pediatric interviewing: a practical, relationship-based approach. New York, NY: Humana Press; 2010.

10. Bryan CJ, Rudd MD. Managing suicide risk in primary care. New York, NY: Springer; 2011.

11. Shea SC, Barney C. Macrotraining: a "how-to" primer for using serial role-playing to train complex clinical interviewing tasks such as suicide assessment. Psychiatr Clin North Am. 2007;30:e1–29.

12. Bryan CJ. Empirically-based outpatient treatment for a patient at risk for suicide: the case of "John". Pragmatic Case Studies Psychother. 2007;3:1–40. http://pcsp.libraries.rutgers.edu.

13. Joiner TE, Steer RA, Brown G, Beck AT, Pettit JW, Rudd MD. Worst-point suicidal plans: a dimension of suicidality predictive of past suicide attempts and eventual death by suicide. Behav Res Ther. 2003;41:1469–80.

14. Berman AL, Jobes DA, Silverman MM. Adolescent suicide: assessment and intervention. Washington, DC: American Psychological Association; 2006.

15. Bryan CJ, Stone SL, Rudd MD. A practical, evidence-based approach for means restriction counseling with suicidal patients. Prof Psychol Res Pr. 2011;42:339–46.

16. McDaniel SH, Campbell TL, Hepworth J, Lorenz A. Family-oriented primary care. 2nd ed. New York, NY: Springer; 2005.

17. Rudd MD, Cordero L, Bryan CJ. What every psychologist should know about the Food and Drug Administration's black box warning label for antidepressants. Prof Psychol Res Pr. 2009;40:321–6.

18. Katz LY, Kozyrskyj AL, Prior HJ, Enns MW, Cox BJ, Sareen J. Effect of regulatory warnings on antidepressant prescription rates, use of health services and outcomes among children, adolescents, and young adults. Can Med Assoc J. 2008;178:1005–11.

Chapter 17
Sex

Role Play

The following basic interviewing tools are prerequisites to participating in role plays for inquiring about sex: *Open-ended inquiries*, *eliciting and responding to feelings*, *self-awareness*, *uncovering health beliefs*, *persistence and clarification*, *transitional statements*, *and normalization*.

Role Play: A 54 yr. old man has COPD. He works part-time. He has poor exercise tolerance. He has been married for 10 years to his second wife.

Objectives

1. Create the context to ask about sexual functioning.
2. Persist when given vague answers.

Trainee	Mr. Stewart, I have a number of questions I would like to ask you about your overall health.
Patient	Okay.
Trainee	Stop me if you have any of the following: headaches, trouble with your vision, hearing problems
Patient	(*interrupts*) My hearing is failing.

(continued)

The online version of this chapter (doi:10.1007/978-1-4614-7224-7_17) contains supplementary material, which is available to authorized users.

Trainee	We'll check that out before you leave today. How about any difficulty swallowing, chest pain, abdominal pain?
Patient	No trouble there.
Trainee	How about with your urine—any blood in the urine, hesitancy or trouble urinating?
Patient	No.
Trainee	Part of my learning about your overall health includes questions about sex. I would like to ask you a few questions to check that out.
Patient	Sure.
Trainee	Are you sexually active?
Patient	Not like I would like to be.
Trainee	That's got to be difficult. Lots of folks with chronic illnesses, like COPD, find they cannot function like they used to. Is that true for you?
Patient	Sometimes I just can't perform the way I used to.
Trainee	Well, even if it is not a frequent problem, we might be able to help.
Patient	Okay.

Feedback

Faculty	Okay. Let's stop. Before, we give you feedback, how did you feel doing the interview?
Trainee	At first, I felt a little awkward, but not too bad.
Faculty	People have affirmations?
Trainee #2	I thought you did a good job. You didn't look tense to me.
Faculty	What did you observe to let you know the interviewer was not tense?
Trainee #2	(to trainee) Your face and body appeared to be relaxed.
Faculty	Anybody else have affirmations?
Trainee #3	You used the third-person technique, "Lots of people with COPD have problems…"
Faculty	I agree. I like the way you set the stage with the review of systems. I like your statement: "Stop me if you had any of the following." You then used a nice transition statement to introduce your inquiries into sexual behavior. Finally, you normalized problems regarding sexual functioning and chronic illness.

(continued)

Trainee	Thanks.
Faculty	Does anybody have options?
Trainee #3	Maybe you could have asked him to tell you what he meant by, "Not like I would like to be." That might give you more information.
Faculty	Good point. Once you know all the specifics about the sexual problem you will be in a better position to make a good diagnosis and help him. It also might be a time to inquire what it has been like for him. He might have a lot of feelings about the changes in his body that you could have explored before empathizing with him? What do you think?
Trainee	I agree. I felt a little nervous at that point and sort of rushed through.
Faculty	Nice awareness. How about replaying from the point you ask him about his sexual activity. This time, stay in there until you know specifics about his sexual functioning. Start from the point you ask him about his functioning

Replay

Trainee	Lots of folks with chronic illnesses, like COPD, find they cannot function sexually like they used to. Is that true for you?
Patient	Some of the time.
Trainee	Say more about that.
Patient	It is just that it can take a while to get an erection, or it might not happen at all.
Trainee	I think we will be able to help you with that. (*trainee stops the interview*)

Feedback

Faculty	(*to trainee*) What are you experiencing?
Trainee	I still feel awkward asking for specific information.
Faculty	Let's talk about feeling awkward. What are you thinking to make yourself feel awkward?

(continued)

Trainee	What do you mean?
Faculty	Some people have beliefs about the elderly, such as they don't need or want accurate information about sexual functioning. Beliefs like that can get in the way of being fully present to the patient when asking about sex.
Trainee	Actually, I partially believe that.
Faculty	What is your belief?
Trainee	I figure that older people rather keep their sexual behavior private. In addition, they probably have all the knowledge they need.
Faculty	Actually, empirical studies don't support that belief. Even though they may have a lot of experience, they frequently have misperceptions about sexual functioning.
Trainee	That's interesting. I will keep that in mind.

Obstacles to Teaching Interviewing About Sex

1. Interviewer is reluctant to bring up sensitive matters, fearful of patient reaction.
2. Interviewer does not follow up on vague answers because of anxiety and avoidance.
3. Interviewer is unaware of self-thoughts that block a full exploration of the sexual history.
4. Taking a sexual history triggers feelings in clinician that are uncomfortable.

Strategies

1. Remind trainee that patients rarely react in a negative way. They expect a sexual history to be part of good health care.
2. Teach trainees to be precise and persistent. Have them repeat role plays in which they did not follow up on vague answers.
3. Initiate a discussion of potential blocking cognitions of clinicians before role playing. Ask participants if they hold any such beliefs.
4. Debrief in a group setting to help trainee with his or her uncomfortable feelings.

Sex

Patients seldom bring up the topic of sex during a primary care visit. Since patients frequently have sexual concerns, it is the responsibility of clinicians to initiate the discussion [1]. Sex is health related. Clinicians must learn to ask about sexual behaviors that place their patients at risk of health problems. As with any sensitive topic, the more a clinician practices, the more natural will be his or her approach. Practice is made easier with the use of a simple structure.

1. Self-examination for thoughts that might interfere with asking patients about sexual behaviors.
2. Create the context to bring up the topic of sex. This allows the clinician to avoid the awkwardness of bringing up a sensitive topic "out of the blue," which can disengage a patient and result in data omission errors. Move to the topic of sexuality with a transition statement.

Self-examination for Interfering Cognitions

The clinician performs a self-examination, scanning for any hidden cognitive blocks to a full, nonjudgmental assessment. For example, a young physician might think: *It is inappropriate to take a sexual history from an adolescent of the opposite sex who is not that much different in age.* The clinician might worry that he or she will appear intrusive and that the patient will react negatively. If the clinician does not stay aware, address, and resolve this issue, he or she might rush the pace or even appear mechanical to the patient. The patient, sensing the clinician's discomfort, will not produce a full and accurate history. That young clinician must stay aware of the fact that good comprehensive care includes a sexual history. The physician–patient relationship forms a professional relationship, not a romantic one. The clinician maintains a clear boundary. The clinician moves to the second step, *setting the stage*, after resolving any internal blocks, such as the one just mentioned.

Another clinician, like the one in the above role play, might hold the following belief: *The elderly don't need or want information about what is normal sexual functioning.* Again, a clinician's first task is to do a self-check for incorrect beliefs and address them (e.g., empirical evidence supports the following statement: the elderly do appreciate appropriate information about sexual functioning [2].)

Setting the Stage

The second step, creating the context to ask about sex, involves two elements:

1. Tell the patient what you would like to do and why you want to do it [3].

| **Clinician** | As your physician, I am interested in all aspects of your health. Because sexuality is connected with a number of important health problems, I ask all my patients a few questions about sex. |

2. Ask permission and obtain their agreement.

| **Clinician** | Is that okay with you? |
| **Patient** | Sure |

An adult sexual history includes sexual behaviors that place patients at risk of health problems and sexual functioning [3]. Many clinicians use the psychosocial history or the genitourinary review of systems as an opportunity to screen for health issues related to sexuality [2, 4]. Frankel et al. recommend screening with the following questions [4]:

Is there someone special in your life? Are you and this person having sex?
Are you satisfied with your sex life? Are there any problems or concerns about your sexual functioning that you'd like to discuss?
Do you have other sexual partners?
It's important that I ask some questions to assess your risk of sexually transmitted diseases or HIV. Have you been having any high risk sex (injection drug users, cocaine users, prostitutes, gay or bisexual men)?
Has your illness affected your sexual functioning?

It is important that the clinician fully explore positive responses and avoid rushing. A biopsychosocial orientation is maintained since relationship issues commonly coexist with sexual problems [5]. For example, chronic medical conditions and surgery can impact patients' self-esteem and sense of attractiveness [4]. Asking them about the impact of the illness on their self-image and sense of self is an important dimension of a sexual history. A guiding, as opposed to a directing, technique allows the clinician to sensitively discuss sexual issues and assess high-risk behaviors, as in the following interview (which is based on the work of Rollnick et. al. in Motivational Interviewing) [6].

A 27-year-old man with a sexually transmitted disease is treated for the condition, followed by brief counseling about STDs, including HIV.

Clinician	The infection you have, gonorrhea, is best treated with an injection of an antibiotic. We will give it to you in a few minutes. Before we do that I would like to talk to you about preventing this type of infection, as well as other risks to your health, in the future. I see that as part of my job. Would that be ok with you?
Patient	What do you mean?
Clinician	It would be important for us to talk about sexually transmitted diseases, including HIV.
Patient	You think I might have HIV?
Clinician	I don't know. I would like to discuss it and ask you questions about risk factors?
Patient	I'm not gay.
Clinician	That is one risk factor. Before we discuss it further, would you be willing to discuss with me how to prevent these types of infections in the future?
Patient	Yes.
Clinician	It would help me if I understood what you already know about HIV and how people get it.
Patient	I know you get it from having sex. And, that it is very serious. I also know that some people live a long time with it, like Magic Johnson.
Clinician	That's correct. We have better ways of treating people with medications when we discover it early. Do you know ways that you can protect yourself from getting HIV?
Patient	I know using condoms prevents HIV.
Clinician	That's right. They work pretty well. How often do you use condoms?
Patient	I am not sure.
Clinician	If you had to guess, what percentage of the time do you use them?
Patient	I would say at least half of the time. I can't always plan.
Clinician	Let me see if I understand correctly. You know that condoms can prevent HIV and you use the half the time. You can't always plan. It is good that you are using condoms. I do have one concern. Could I share it with you?
Patient	Yes.
Clinician	We know that HIV can be spread with just one sexual encounter, even from somebody that is healthy and does not even look sick.
Patient	Maybe I should be more careful about using condoms.

(continued)

Clinician	Using condoms all the time would decrease your risk, as well as your partner's risk. What do you think of that recommendation?
Patient	I think it sounds like a good idea.
Clinician	Will you commit to it?
Patient	I will. I wonder if I already could have HIV
Clinician	We could test for that today. What do you say?
Patient	It's scary to think that.
Clinician	I imagine it is very frightening to think you might have a positive test.
Patient	Yes. However, it would be better to know.
Clinician	The other question that would be important to talk about is the number of partners you have had.
Patient	Several.
Clinician	Would you be more specific?
Patient	I had a girlfriend for a several years until we broke up 6 weeks ago. I never cheated. Since then I have had sex with one woman, one time.
Clinician	Did you use a condom with that encounter?
Patient	No.
Clinician	Let me summarize what you have told me to make sure we are on the same page… You understand that HIV is a serious condition. It can often be treated effectively when it is diagnosed early. It can be spread from people who look healthy. Using condoms all the time can prevent HIV, although not 100 percent of the time. You will get tested today and come back in a couple of days for me to discuss the results with you. It might be good for us to talk about your partners when you come back. How does that sound to you?
Patient	Sounds ok to me.
Clinician	Just to make sure we are on same page, would you say back to me what our plan is?
Patient	I need to use condoms every time to have the best chance to prevent HIV. You are going to send me for HIV testing and I will come back next week to talk with you about it.
Comment	*When the patient returns to discuss results and his partner relationships, it will be important to inquire about his emotions. People often have feelings of fear, shame, and guilt related to sexually transmitted diseases* [4].

The basic structure outlined above gives the novice an interviewing strategy to smoothly introduce and then discuss sex. Adolescents are at a unique stage of their life cycle and sexual development [7]. The above approach needs to be modified for them.

Adolescent Sexuality

Adolescents are in the midst of figuring out who they are. Sexuality is an important aspect of their emerging sense of self. Since that identity is not yet solidly established, they can be more sensitive to a parental or condescending tone of voice [4]. It can be helpful to begin with nonthreatening, closed-ended questions. They frequently need more time to talk about nonsensitive issues (set the stage), before they feel comfortable discussing sex. They will discuss sensitive topics with their physician only when they trust the *confidentiality* of their revelations. Typically a primary care physician will talk to children without parents present for part of the visit, starting during the preteen years. Privacy is discussed with the family then and repeated as appropriate. A clear confidentiality *contract* helps the family understand the clinical rationale underlying the request for privacy [8].

Clinician	Ben, now that you are older and can take more responsibility for keeping yourself healthy, it is important that we talk about how the visits will go. As your doctor, I am the person you see when you have sore throats and coughs. I am also interested in you as a whole person. And, I know that teenagers face all kinds of decisions about personal things that can really affect their health—things like sex, stress, depression, alcohol, and drugs [9]. I am going to ask you questions about those things because I want to help you make the best decisions in taking care of your health. I know these topics are usually private and can be hard to talk about. I will not tell your parents or anyone else what you tell me. The only exception is a situation in which your life or someone else's life was in immediate danger. For example, if you were planning on killing yourself. In that case, I would talk to your parents to find ways to help you. My goal is to help you be healthy. I can best do that if you are open and honest with me. Is this agreeable with you, Ben?
Patient	Yes, it is.

Set the Stage

Once contracting is complete, the clinician transitions to questions about home and school. Adolescents typically answer these questions freely, which allows for later movement to sensitive areas. This clinician sets the stage by asking about friends.

Clinician	Tell me about your friendships at school.
Patient	I've got several really good friends.
Clinician	(*echoing*) You've got several really good friends.
Patient	Yeah. We all hang out at lunchtime. We eat at the same table.
Clinician	Do you see your friends outside of school?
Patient	We're always together.
Clinician	What do you like to do for fun?
Patient	Lots of times we just talk.
Clinician	It sounds like your friendships are a high priority in your life.
Patient	That's true.
Clinician	Lots of teenagers your age are beginning to have romantic relationships. Is that true for you?
Patient	Yes. I've been talking to someone.

Normalization

The clinician then uses the third-person technique during the conversation about friendships and romantic relationships to smoothly transition to the topic of sexuality. The discussion of friends and romantic relationships operates as a gateway to sexuality. The transition to a discussion of sexuality feels natural and normal to the patient, as in the following example: *Some folks in high school are starting to have an interest in boys or girls in a sexual way* [10]. *Is that true for you?* The clinician avoids confusion by avoiding asking if the adolescent is sexually active. Many adolescents interpret "sexually active" in ways that were not intended by the interviewer [11]. In addition, the above questioning does not make assumptions about sexual orientation. A gay or lesbian adolescent is then more likely to open up to the clinician.

The clinician tracks with the patient's answers. If the teenager is having sex, the clinician can ask about partners, the use of protection from pregnancy and sexually transmitted diseases, and the presence of violence in the relationship. The third-person technique is helpful when introducing the topic of violence (without the partner present):

Clinician	Violence is so common among the young people I see in my practice I ask all of them the following question "Have you been pushed, slapped, hurt, or forced to have sex by anyone with whom you live or are close to?" [12]
Patient	No.

Teenagers not having sex can be asked how they feel about that and affirmed for their decision. They can be offered the opportunity to discuss these topics whenever the teenager is ready to take in that information.

Key Points

1. The context for talking with adolescents about sex is established with a clear contract for what will be discussed during the visit.
2. It is often helpful to begin the discussion of sexuality with adolescents on less sensitive topics.
3. An adult sexual history involves asking about high-risk sexual behaviors and problems with functioning.
4. Clarify vague answers.
5. It is important to consider the relationship dynamics.
6. Remember to inquire about vulnerable feelings, such as fear, shame, and guilt, and support the patient's feelings.

References

1. Epstein RM, Morse DS, Frankel RM, Frarey L, Anderson K, Beckman HB. Awkward moments in patient-physician communication about HIV risk. Ann Intern Med. 1998;128:435–47.
2. Ende J, Rockwell S, Glasgow M. The sexual history in general medical practice. Arch Intern Med. 1984;144:558–61.
3. Platt FW, Gordon GH. Field guide to the difficult patient interview. 2nd ed. Williams and Wilkins, PA: Lippincott; 2004.
4. Frankel RM, Williams S, Edwardsen E. Asking about sexuality. In: Novack DH, Clark WD, Daetwyler C, Saizow DB, editors. doc.com – an interactive learning resource for healthcare communication [Internet]. Philadelphia, PA: American Academy on Communication in Healthcare/Drexel University College of Medicine. Accessed 10 May 2012. http://www.AACHonline.org.
5. Williams S. The sexual history. In: Lipkin M, Putnam S, Lazare A, editors. The medical interview: clinical care education and research. New York, NY: Springer; 1995.
6. Rollnick S, Miller WR, Butler CC. Motivational interviewing in health care: helping patients change behavior. New York, NY: The Guilford Press; 2008.
7. Lief HI, Berman EM. Sexual interviewing throughout the patient's cycle. In: Lief HI, editor. Sexual problems in medical practice. Chicago, IL: American Medical Association; 1981.
8. Ginsberg K. The adolescent interview. In: Novack DH, Clark WD, Daetwyler C, Saizow DB, editors. doc.com – an interactive learning resource for healthcare communication [Internet]. Philadelphia, PA: American Academy on Communication in healthcare/Drexel University College of Medicine. Accessed 17 Mar 2012. http://www.AACHonline.org.
9. Millstein S, Irwin C, Adler N, Cohn L, Kegeles S, Dolcini M. Health-risk behaviors and health concerns among young adolescents. Pediatrics. 1992;89:422–8.
10. Maehr J, Felice M. Eleven to fourteen years: early adolescence age of rapid changes. In: Dixon SD, Stein MT, editors. Encounters with children: pediatric behavior and development. 4th ed. Philadelphia, PA: Mosby Elsevier; 2006.

11. Maehr J, Felice M. Fifteen to seventeen years: mid adolescence – redefining self. In: Dixon SD, Stein MT, editors. Encounters with children: pediatric behavior and development. 4th ed. Philadelphia, PA: Mosby Elsevier; 2006.
12. Little KJ. Screening for domestic violence: identifying, assisting, and empowering adult victims of abuse. Postgrad Med. 2000;108:135–41.

Chapter 18
Motivational Interviewing

Role Play

Prerequisite skills that need to be mastered before role-playing motivational interviewing with patients regarding alcohol use include *self-awareness, contracting, personal story, open-ended inquiries, facilitatory gestures, empathic summaries*, and *third-person technique*. It is particularly important that trainees have previously practiced empathetic summaries to a level of competence.

Role Play #1:   The patient is a 42-year-old homeless male in the ER for evaluation of minor head trauma.

Objectives

1. Use a transition statement to move to the area of substance abuse.
2. Screen for alcohol use problems.

Trainee	Mr. Riley, lots of times when people have had a fall and hit their head, we find that is important to ask about the use of alcohol and drugs. Would that be okay with you?
Patient	I don't do any drugs.
Trainee	How about alcohol?
Patient	I have two beers a day, sometimes three.
Trainee	So you have two to three beers a day.
Patient	That's all I can afford.
Trainee	What size are the beers?
Patient	I buy the 40 ounce ones.

(continued)

J. Binder, *Primary Care Interviewing: Learning Through Role Play*,
DOI 10.1007/978-1-4614-7224-7_18, © Springer Science+Business Media New York 2013

Trainee	Is it okay if I ask you a few more questions about drinking?
Patient	Sure.
Faculty	Let's stop there. You met the objectives of the role play. You used the third- person techniques to introduce the topic and then initiated a screen for alcohol use problems. I like the way you clarified the size of the beers. It was important information, which would need to be explored further. Nice job.

Role Play #2:   This is a 48-year-old woman recently hospitalized with acute hepatitis secondary to alcohol abuse.

Objectives

1. Assess the impact of patient's drinking on patient's life.
2. Present the diagnosis of alcohol abuse to the patient in a caring, nonconfrontational manner.

Trainee	I would like to ask you some questions about how your drinking might be affecting your life in other areas besides the recent bout with hepatitis.
Patient	Okay.
Trainee	Tell me about your personal life.
Patient	I am recently divorced and have two daughters, 11 and 14. I am doing substitute teaching after being a stay-at-home mother for several years.
Trainee	So, you have gone through a divorce and started a new job. It sounds difficult.
Patient	It is.
Trainee	Has that triggered more drinking?
Patient	A little bit, but I have not had a drink since I got out of the hospital.
Trainee	Good for you.
Patient	Thanks.
Trainee	How do you think alcohol has affected you in terms of holding up your day-to-day responsibilities?
Patient	I don't think it has affected that. I have not missed any work, except when I was in the hospital.
Trainee	How about your relationships?
Patient	My ex-husband might say that it caused problems in our relationship.

(continued)

Trainee	What do you think?
Patient	We both drank. It was part of our problem.
Trainee	How about any other relationships?
Patient	No.
Trainee	Let me summarize. You have had health problems, the hepatitis, as well as problems in one relationship secondary to the drinking. We call that alcohol abuse.
Patient	I don't think I abuse alcohol. I might drink a little much now because of the stress I'm under.
Trainee	I'm just giving you the medical diagnosis we use for this situation.
Patient	It makes me sound pretty bad.
Trainee	I'm not trying to make you sound bad.

Feedback

Faculty	Okay, Let's stop. (*to trainee*) What are you experiencing?
Trainee	I am a little confused. I am not sure where to go with her answer.
Faculty	Say more about that.
Trainee	She seems annoyed with the diagnosis. I'm not sure what to say to her.
Faculty	Let's come back to that. Do people have affirmations?
Trainee #2	I thought you did a really good job of finding out about the effects on her personal life.
Patient	I thought it was important to tell me upfront that you were going to be asking about the effects of alcohol in my life.
Trainee #3	I liked the way you asked her to tell you her personal story.
Faculty	I agree with all the above. In addition, I thought you showed good self-awareness. People with alcohol problems can often trigger defensive feelings in the clinician. Patients like this one can minimize their condition.
Trainee	Thank you.
Faculty	I have one or two options of responding in this type of situation.
Trainee	I would like suggestions. She definitely seemed upset when I mentioned alcohol abuse.
Faculty	When she became upset, I might just reflect back what she is saying and feeling, "So, you see yourself as a social drinker

(continued)

	and seem a little surprised I used the words alcohol abuse. Is that right?" In other words, you don't struggle. You roll with the resistance. One of the keys to managing a difficult interaction successfully is to recognize the moment something goes wrong, such as, "It makes me sound pretty bad."
Trainee	How could I talk to her about the diagnosis and recommendations?
Faculty	The elicit-provide-elicit structure works well in this situation. You ask the patient what her perspective is and then give information in small chunks. "I notice you seemed quiet when I used the word 'alcohol abuse.' It is a technical term. It sounds like we might have a different understanding of that term. The important thing is for us to be able to talk about the situation together. Is that okay with you?"
Trainee	I could see how that approach would help. It would be a relief to not believe that I had to get her to accept my diagnosis of alcohol abuse.
Faculty	Right. And, it is a way to support autonomy. Are you ready to do replay the situation?
Trainee	Yes.

Replay

Trainee	I would like to ask you some questions about how your drinking might be affecting your life.
Patient	Okay.
Trainee	Would you start by telling me about your personal life.
Patient	I am recently divorced and have two daughters, 11 and 14. I had not worked for several years, but I recently started doing substitute teaching.
Trainee	It sounds stressful.
Patient	It is.
Trainee	Has that triggered more drinking?
Patient	Maybe a little bit, but I have not had a drink since I got out of the hospital.
Trainee	That's very good. How did you decide to do make that change?
Patient	I wasn't feeling very well.
Trainee	Is giving up alcohol a decision you would consider making permanent at this point? That would be my recommendation for anybody that has alcohol abuse.
Patient	I don't abuse alcohol. That sounds very bad.

(continued)

> **Trainee**   Labeling the drinking as alcohol abuse sounds bad, perhaps like a criticism... Let me summarize where we are. I suggested that you stop drinking totally because of my diagnosis of alcohol abuse. You seemed surprised that I called it alcohol abuse—almost as if I blindsided you. You consider the problem to be less serious.
>
> **Patient**   I am surprised. I am not angry.
>
> **Trainee**   Thank you for saying that. Sometimes, we use terms that sound uncomplimentary. Would you be willing to do talk more about where we go from here?

Feedback

> **Faculty**   Let's stop. You accomplished what we discussed. You gave her the diagnosis and then rolled with the resistance. You summarized her thoughts and feelings in an empathic manner and attempted to find common ground. Nice job....

Obstacles to Teaching Motivational Interviewing

1. Interviewer has a tendency to rescue or take responsibility for the other person.
2. Interviewer has a deeply held belief that substance abusers will not change.
3. Interviewer is concerned that talking with patients about lifestyle changes will take too much time.

Strategies

1. Teach trainees about the destructive impact of rescuing others, even though the motivation is caring.
2. Show trainees data that office interventions can be successful with substance abusers.
3. Discuss the effectiveness of using brief and repeated interviews in the office. Interventions with family members can be scheduled for longer visits.

Motivational Interviewing

A second-year pediatric resident enters the conference room, announcing she just examined a child whose mother smoked in the presence of her child, despite his diagnosis of asthma. The resident wants to give the mother a "piece of my mind."

This brief scenario highlights not one, but two, separate myths regarding behavioral changes.

Myth #1:   People change behaviors when they are confronted, scolded, or persuaded with repeated explanations of the problem [1].

Myth #2:   The clinician is responsible for changing a patient's behavior, rather than helping the patient realize his or her own resources and reasons for changing [1].

Confrontation and attempts to persuade patients with repeated explanations result from a basic misunderstanding of how people change lifestyle behaviors, such as overeating, drinking, or not exercising. People are more likely to make an internal change when they view themselves as capable and basically okay people—not when they are experiencing shame, humiliation, or fear. Fear may work in the short term, but does not provide the support that leads to lasting change. Sustained change results from a patient making a personal commitment to him or herself. The patient must believe that he or she is capable of changing and that change would be beneficial. The tasks of the clinician, then, are to understand the patient's feelings, beliefs, and priorities and elicit change-talk from the patient that will help the patient align his or her behavior with deeply held values [1]. It is the patient's reasons for change, not the clinician's, which will drive long-lasting change. Changing to please someone else does not work. Motivational interviewing is a tool that clinicians can use to help patients and families find their own resources to make lifestyle changes.

In this chapter, motivational interviewing principles will be described in the context of screening, assessing, and intervening with adult patients who have alcohol use problems. It is an introduction to motivational interviewing in primary care. The skills to become proficient are not acquired in one or two role plays. Ongoing supervision and mentoring are required. Empirical evidence supports the benefit of learning these skills. Motivational interviewing is effective, even in the brief interventions characteristic of medical office visits [1, 2]. Since 50 % of the mortality in primary care results from lifestyle behaviors, any tool that can impact those factors is important [3]. The clinician also benefits. **The principle of respect for a patient's autonomy, inherent in the motivational interviewing approach, allows the clinician to avoid the stress and depletion that is an inevitable consequence of believing one is responsible for changing another person's behavior.** It is helpful for clinicians to stay aware that most patients are ambivalent about changing. Patients are more likely to move in a positive direction if the clinician uses the principles of motivational interviewing. However, some patients will not be ready to change. Understanding and accepting those patients may encourage them to change in the future [4].

Motivational Interviewing with Alcohol Use Disorders

The majority of patients with alcohol use disorders are not identified in primary care [5]. Sensitive and reliable questionnaires are readily available. The U.S. Preventive Services Task Force recommends screening all adult patients [6]. The three-part interviewing structure previously discussed with other sensitive issues is applicable (see Chap. 16).

Self-examination

The clinician performs a self-examination for any thoughts or feelings that might block adopting a nonjudgmental, caring approach to patients with alcohol use disorders. These patients commonly act defensive, sometimes aggressively, minimize their symptoms, or give vague responses, all of which can trigger frustration and helplessness in clinicians. It is important for the clinician not to adopt a helpless stance with these patients since one-third of them make significant changes with intervention [7]. Much harm can be prevented.

The clinician can resolve the problem of defensiveness by staying self-aware and reminding him or herself of the effectiveness of motivational interviewing, even when patients are defensive. A clinician staying fully self-aware will also attend to any current emotional reactions to his or her patients with alcohol problems and related family-of-origin experiences.

Set the Stage

Learning about the patient as a person and engaging with the patient are the most critical steps in setting the stage [8]. Once engaged, the clinician moves to an inquiry into alcohol use with a transition statement, explaining the reason for asking about high-risk health behaviors [8]. An example might be: *I am interested in the overall health of my patients—the sore throats, the stresses they face, as well as lifestyle behaviors that have a big impact on health, such as alcohol use.* Alternatively, the clinician can use a normalizing statement like: *I ask all my patients about alcohol use because of its importance in health outcomes Do you drink alcoholic beverages?*

Assessment

Patients with a positive screen are assessed for alcohol use disorders, a continuum that runs from high-risk drinking to alcohol dependence.

High-risk drinking behavior needs to be assessed.

- *Do you drive after drinking?*
- *How many times in the past year have you had five or more drinks?* (four or more for women). These are limits set by the National Institute on Alcohol Abuse (NIAAA). Weekly limits set by the NIAAA are 14 drinks for men and 7 drinks for women and those over 65. A drink is one 12-oz beer or equivalent [9].

Alcohol abuse and dependence are diagnosed by obtaining details about the impact of drinking on relationships, role responsibilities at home and work, legal problems, and high-risk drinking [9, 10]. Alcohol dependence is diagnosed when multiple medical and psychosocial problems are present, with or without physical dependence [11]. The CAGE questions were initially designed to screen for alcohol dependence but are frequently used to ease the movement of the conversation to the topic of drinking [10].

CAGE

- *Have you ever felt that you should cut down on your drinking?*
- *Have people annoyed you by criticizing your drinking?*
- *Have you ever felt bad or guilty about your drinking?*
- *Have you ever had a drink first thing in the morning to steady your nerves or get rid of a hangover (eye opener)?*

Validity

Since patients frequently minimize and even lie about their drinking, it is important to adopt interviewing strategies to increase accuracy.

1. One technique that sidesteps the tendency of the patient to minimize is to ask for other people's opinions. *What would your wife say about the effect of your drinking on your relationship with her?*
2. Gentle assumption is a technique that assumes the behavior is occurring [12]. *How often do you have five or more drinks?* This makes it more difficult for a patient to deny the behavior.
3. Another validity technique, denial of the specific, is based on the principle that a patient has more difficulty lying about a behavior when he or she is asked directly about the behavior in question [12]. *Do you smoke marijuana?* (See Chap. 8 for further development of gentle assumption and denial of the specific.)
4. Focused questions, like those above, often work better during this phase of the interview. Open-ended questions can lead to vague answers and create tension and suspiciousness as the clinician attempts to clarify the answer [11]. And, as noted previously, the key to interviewing patients with alcohol use disorders is maintaining a strong engagement. If the interviewer senses irritation with a question, he or she can make the resistance overt [11]. *I hear some concern in your voice. Let me explain why I am asking these questions.*

Complete the Assessment

Alcohol abuse and dependence should be diagnosed and common coexisting conditions identified (e.g., use of other medications, use of alcohol before driving, depression, anxiety) [13]. Standardized interviews, such as the Alcohol Use

Disorders Identification Test (AUDIT), can help [13]. Part of that assessment should include an inquiry regarding tolerance and withdrawal [10]:

Have you noticed that you must drink more to get the same effect?
In the early afternoon, before you start any drinking, do you notice any shakiness or nervousness that goes away once you start drinking?

However, the clinician does not need to obtain every detail before intervening, since the initial interventions will be similar for most patients [11]. In addition, repeated short interventions are a good fit for the primary care model.

Brief Interventions[1] in Alcohol Use Disorders

Brief interventions, lasting 10–15 min, have been shown to reduce high-risk drinking [2, 13]. A large body of evidence supports effectiveness of motivational interviewing, even when patients don't appear to be ready for change [1, 15]. In fact, 75 % of patients do have some readiness to change [15]. The following four strategies are integral to a motivational interviewing approach [1].

Use the Elicit–Provide–Elicit Framework for Giving Information

Elicit: The clinician seeks out the patient's perspective, understanding of the condition, values, and his other priorities; also, he or she does not judge or correct that perspective [1]. *Tell me the importance of your friendships and the role drinking plays in those friendships.*
Provide: Information is given in small chunks. Facts, not judgments or opinions (*Alcohol is destroying your life*), are given [11]. A clinician might make any of the following brief statements:

- *Tremors and feeling nervous after a period of not drinking are signs that drinking has affected brain cells and changed the way they function.*
- *Problem drinking can sneak up on people.*
- *Your wife says that your marriage is going poorly and that your drinking is a problem.*

Elicit: When a recommendation is made or a patient reacts nonverbally to a statement, the clinician checks it out [10]. *I notice you seemed quiet after I said your diagnosis is alcohol abuse. Tell me what you think about what I said.*

---

[1] Adapted with permission from Clark and Parish [14].

Roll with the Resistance

A clinician adjusts his or her response depending on the patient's readiness to change. For a patient not very interested in changing, the clinician simply reflects back the patient's position [1]. *Currently, you do not see that your drinking is a problem. I have a different perspective than you. I am concerned about the effects of drinking on your health and would like to bring the issue up in the future. Is that okay with you?* Many patients are ambivalent about their drinking. It is important for the clinician to not push on the side of changing, since this typically leads to increased resistance [1]. Acknowledging the ambivalence and helping the patient voice the pros and cons of changing, or not changing, leave the responsibility for managing the ambivalence with the patient.

Clinician	**A part of you** sees clear advantages to becoming sober. You would feel physically better. You have had a lot of stomach problems that have been worsened by the drinking. You acknowledge problems in your relationship with your fiancée, who wants you to stop drinking. Most important of all, you feel bad about yourself after you binge. On the other hand, you highly value your drinking friendships. Your drinking friends have been your buddies since grade school and they always drink when you get together. You would feel like an outsider if you stopped drinking. You also like to party and the feeling when you drink. Do I have it correct?
Patient	Yes. That's basically it.

The art is in helping the patient develop his or her own motivation to close the gap between actual and desired ways of behaving. Some patients will not have a strong motivation to obtain symptom relief. The following two inquiries can help these patients access other motivations for change:

- *Is there anything that your alcohol use keeps you from doing that you would really like to do again (lost dreams)?*
- *Are there family members for whom you want to stay healthy in order to take care of them?* [16]

Support Change

Primary care patients commonly change after a series of brief interventions, in which the clinician carefully tracks the patient's process [2]. The patient is asked to expand on any spontaneous change-talk, such as: *Tell me more about your thought of cutting back on your drinking, if you can find another way to deal with the stress.* Resistance talk is simply reflected back. *Your friends all drink and your social life is organized around drinking.* Information is provided using the elicit–provide–elicit (EPE) format. It is often helpful to ask permission to give the patient facts or information: *Would it be okay if I share what we have learned about abstinence and drinking friendships?* Tracking carefully with the patient increases engagement and decreases resistance.

Assessment of the patient's level of motivation and confidence to make a change, and why he or she is at those levels, help guide the clinician during the change process [17]. Keller and Kemp-White suggest the following questions:

- *How important is this behavior change to you, on a scale of one to ten?*
- *How confident are you that you can make this change, on a scale of one to ten?*
- *Tell me why you rated them like you did.*

This information is used to plan the next step. "A patient who is unconvinced may need to see data. A convinced, but unconfident, patient may need help planning simple steps toward change." [8, p. 80].

Give Specific Recommendations Congruent with Expert Guidelines

Abstinence should be advised for alcohol abuse and dependence. Patient agreement with the plan is sought by giving a clear rationale based on the empirical evidence [11]. It is important to negotiate a plan of action, even if a very small step, one that all parties agree to follow.

Clinician	You acknowledge that your drinking has affected several important relationships in your life. Your efforts to cut back have not worked for you in the past. I would recommend abstinence and that you attend three different AA meetings this week and try them out. AA members can give you the support you have not had in the past. What do you think of that suggestion?
Patient	It might be worth a try. I certainly have not been able to do it on my own.

Patients need a lot of external support, education, and coaching during early recovery. Changing their basic ways of surviving and adapting can be frightening and overwhelming [18]. Referral for specialized treatment is recommended for all patients with significant adverse consequences of using alcohol [9]. The family needs support as well. Recovery from alcohol addiction affects the entire family. Marital conflict and emotional and behavioral problems with children commonly mark the early years of sobriety [18].

Key Points

1. Adopting healthy lifestyle behaviors is more likely to be sustained when patients align their behavior with their core values.
2. Motivational interviewing can be effective with brief interventions.
3. The basic stance of motivational interviewing is one of empathy and respect for the autonomy of the individual.
4. The elicit–provide–elicit framework is one effective way of counseling lifestyle changes.

References

1. Rollnick S, William WR, Butler CC. Motivational interviewing in health care: helping patients change behavior. New York, NY: The Guilford Press; 2008.
2. Whitlock EP, Polen MR, Green CA, Orleans T, Klein J. Behavioral counseling interventions in primary care to reduce risky/harmful alcohol use by adults: a summary of the evidence of U.S. Preventive Services Task Force. Ann Intern Med. 2004;140:557–68.
3. McGinnis JM, Foege WH. Actual cases of death in the United States. JAMA. 1993;270: 2207–12.
4. Widdowson M. Transactional analysis: 100 key points and techniques. New York, NY: Routledge; 2010.
5. Coulton S, Drummond C, James P, Godfrey C, Bland JM, Parrott S, et al. Opportunistic screening for alcohol use disorders in primary care: comparative study. BMJ. 2006;332:511–7.
6. U.S. Preventive Services Task Force. Screening and behavioral counseling interventions in primary care to reduce alcohol misuse: recommendation statement. Ann Intern Med. 2009;140:554–6.
7. Miller WR, Walters ST, Bennett ME. How effective is alcoholism treatment in the United States. J Stud Alcohol. 2001;62:211–20.
8. Platt FW, Gordon GH. Field guide to the difficult patient interview. 2nd ed. Philadelphia, PA: Lippincott Williams & Wilkins; 2004.
9. National Institute on Alcohol Abuse and Alcoholism (NIAAA). Helping patients who drink too much: a clinician's guide. Washington, DC: GPO; 2005 (NIH, 301-443-3860, http://www.niaaa.nih.gov).
10. Clark W, Parish S. Alcohol interviewing and advising. In: Novack DH, Clark WD, Daetwyler C, Saizow DB, editors. doc.com – an interactive learning resource for healthcare communication [Internet]. Philadelphia, PA: American Academy on Communication in healthcare/Drexel University College of Medicine. Accessed on 21 May 2012. http://www.AACHonline.org.
11. Clark W. Alcohol and substance abuse. In: Feldman M, Christensen J, editors. Behavioral medicine: a guide for clinical practice. New York, NY: McGraw Hill; 2008.
12. Shea SC. Psychiatric interviewing: the art of understanding: a practical guide for psychiatrists, psychologists, counselors, social workers, nurses, and other mental health professionals. 2nd ed. Philadelphia, PA: WB Saunders; 1998.
13. Saitz R. Unhealthy alcohol use. N Engl J Med. 2005;352:596–607.
14. Clark W, Parish S. Alcohol: interviewing and advising. In: Novack DH et al., editors. doc.com – an interactive learning resource for health communication [Internet]. Philadelphia, PA: American Academy on Communication in Healthcare/Drexel University College of Medicine. Accessed 15 Feb 12. http://www.AACHonline.org.

15. Williams EC, Kivlahan DR, Saitz R, Merrill JO, Achtmeyer CE, McCormick KA, et al. Readiness to change in primary care patients who screened positive for alcohol misuse. Ann Fam Med. 2006;4:213–20.
16. Shea SC. Improving medication adherence: how to talk with patients about their medications. New York, NY: Lippincott Williams and Wilkins; 2006.
17. Keller VF, Kemp-White M. Choices and changes: a new model for influencing patient health behavior. J Clin Outcomes Manag. 1997;4:33–6.
18. Brown S, Lewis VM. The alcoholic family in recovery: a developmental model. New York, NY: The Guilford Press; 2002.

Chapter 19
Giving Bad News

Role Play

The following basic skills are prerequisites to role-playing giving bad news: ***attending, listening***, *eliciting feelings, checking patient's **theory of illness**, monitoring pace, **empathic summary, feeling responses**, and **self-awareness***.

Role Play: Stephanie, a 21-year-old education student, is the mother of a 3-year-old boy, Sam. They live with Stephanie's grandmother in a rural area. Stephanie believes Sam has an anger problem. This is their first visit to the pediatric clinic at the hospital center. A screening questionnaire identified language and social deficits. The physical exam was remarkable for markedly delayed language.

Objectives

1. Check mother's understanding of the meaning of the information provided.
2. Elicit mother's feelings.

Trainee	Stephanie, I would like to talk to you about Sam's development as well as his anger.
Mother	Okay.
Trainee	I agree with you that his language is not normal for his age. That may be related to the difficulty he has had learning to manage his anger.
Mother	What can I do about it?

(continued)

J. Binder, *Primary Care Interviewing: Learning Through Role Play*,
DOI 10.1007/978-1-4614-7224-7_19, © Springer Science+Business Media New York 2013

Trainee	Let's talk about that in a minute. First, tell me what you think about my saying his language is not normal.
Mother	I knew he was behind. It's hard to hear someone say it. It makes it real.
Trainee	I imagine it is very difficult to hear Sam's language is behind.
Mother	Yes.
Trainee	I think we should have it checked out, especially since you say he doesn't play well with other children. I know a psychologist who specializes in evaluating young children.
Mother	Does he have autism? I was reading about that on the internet. If he does, I would love him just the same. I would want him to start treatment.
Trainee	I'm not sure what his diagnosis is. I think it would be good to check it out, so you know what you are dealing with.

Feedback

Faculty	(to interviewer) Let's stop. Tell me what you liked about the interview.
Trainee	I felt I addressed her concerns and went at a slow pace. I thought we had good rapport.
Faculty	How about others?
Mother	You made good eye contact and I felt you cared about me.
Trainee #2	It is a challenging situation. I thought you handled it smoothly. That's not easy.
Faculty	Would you tell her how she handled it smoothly?
Trainee #2	You (trainee) told her the situation was difficult and a lot to bear. You talked slowly.
Faculty	I also noticed that you had a soft, warm manner that conveyed empathy. That is so key in this situation. You asked her what she thought about your statement regarding the language development. This allowed you to know what meaning she placed on your statement. How about options?
Trainee #3	I thought it might have been helpful to use an empathetic summary regarding her concern about the anger.
Faculty	My option piggybacks on that theme. I would suggest pausing after you give her a chunk of information or she shares her thoughts about her child. Ask her what she is feeling. You already have a warm, compassionate manner. This would build on that, inviting her to share her feelings. Any time someone

(continued)

	mentions that they have considered a devastating condition like autism, they likely have big underlying feelings. I might say, "What do you feel emotionally as you consider the diagnosis of autism?"
Trainee	She is probably scared and sad.
Faculty	Yes. And, if she shares her feelings with you, I would suggest a feeling response, such as silence or commenting on what a big loss this is for her.
Trainee	That makes good sense to me.
Faculty	Okay. Let's run through it again.

Replay

Trainee	Stephanie, let's talk about your concerns about Sam's anger when things don't go like he wants. This might be related to his difficulty expressing himself in words.
Mother	I do think that is true. I just don't know how to handle him when he gets so angry.
Trainee	That has got to be difficult. I think the first step in helping you is to figure out the cause of his language deficit and how that might be related to his anger problem. You mentioned he has trouble playing with other children.
Mother	I wonder if that is because he does not get much of a chance to play with children.
Trainee	So you think it might be lack of experience?
Mother	Maybe.
Trainee	It is true that experience is important. However, I am concerned it is more than that.
Mother	What do you think it is?
Trainee	I don't know. I do think we need a thorough evaluation. What is it like to hear this?
Mother	I feel sad (*she cries*).
Trainee	(*remains silent and attends to her nonverbally*)… It's a big loss.
Mother	I have read about autism on the internet. Do you think that is what it is?
Trainee	I imagine it is very difficult to even consider that possibility.
Mother	I'll love him no matter what. I want to get him started in treatment if that is the case.
Trainee	Of course.
Mother	I can't believe something is wrong with Sam.

(continued)

Trainee	It sounds like this news is hard to accept.
M0ther	(*continues to be tearful*) Yes, it seems surreal.
Trainee	(*listens attentively in silence*)
Faculty	Let's stop. (*to trainee*) You set the stage, gave her support all along the way, and responded with a warm, feeling response. Wonderful job!

Obstacles to Teaching Giving Bad News

1. Interviewer avoids the vulnerable feelings giving bad news can trigger in the clinician.
2. Interviewer rushes to telling the patient what can be done about the condition.

Strategies

1. Use the role-play group to discuss feelings triggered by giving bad news
2. Learn the difference between thinking and feeling responses to grieving patients

Giving Bad News[1]

Giving bad news to patients in an empathic, thoughtful manner is one of the most important tasks of a clinician. Patients suffer immediate and long-term negative consequences when bad news is delivered poorly [2]. Learning how to be with a patient who is grieving or dying can be a bigger challenge than learning the mechanics of giving bad news, although both are important and intertwined [3]. Staying present to grieving parents is particularly tough. The potential loss of a child is the greatest loss a human can suffer. Parents who lose a child must grieve the loss of all their hopes and dreams for the future of that child, as well as for their own future [4]. I will devote the first part of this chapter to the issue of staying emotionally present to patients and families facing bad news, before looking at expert recommendations for giving bad news.

Staying Emotionally Present to Families

During the Marshall University Department of Pediatrics ongoing interviewing seminar for residents, we looked at the type of thoughts physicians express when faced with giving bad news. Residents endorsed the following concerns during one workshop on giving bad news:

---

[1] Adapted from Binder [1] with permission.

"I might not say the right thing."

"I don't know how to explain everything."

"I might make a mistake that would be terrible."

"I'm inadequate to the task."

"I wouldn't be able to handle it if the family had a huge reaction."

"I don't want them to blame me."

"I won't be able to handle it if they get angry with me."

"I can't deal with the potential loss of a child."

A physician holding any of these beliefs will be distracted. Many of these beliefs reflect **core** beliefs about self in relationship to others. Because negative core beliefs about self are often formed as a result of discouraging or hurtful childhood experiences, they are stored in parts of the brain that become activated by painful feelings, such as anxiety or sadness [5]. Physicians commonly experience these painful feelings when faced with the task of giving bad news and, then, attempt to avoid those painful feelings by busily trying to protect families from feeling bad. Sometimes, this attempt to avoid painful feelings is a reflection of unfinished grief from the clinician's own past, which has been triggered by the family's grief [4].

A brief exploration of several negative core cognitions will demonstrate that they are distorted or inaccurate. A physician who must "say it right" or "know everything" is expressing a euphemism for "I must do it perfectly." In striving to reach that impossible and unreachable standard, the physician is not really able to listen to the patient. Instead, he or she is responding to an internal voice saying "Do it perfectly." [6] Yet, patients do not want perfect doctors. Survey after survey confirms that they want **good enough** doctors who are compassionate. Another statement from the seminar promotes a myth about feelings: "They will have too big an emotional reaction." The idea that feelings the patient expresses might be 'too much' distorts reality. Babies are not born dampening down their feelings. They cry fully to communicate their needs. Only over time do they learn from the environment that certain feelings are too much [7]. Intense feelings are an appropriate expression of grief.

When a clinician is faced with giving bad news, his or her first task is a self-examination for any thoughts or fears that might get in the way of being fully present to the patient or family. Any barriers must be removed. For example, a clinician who realizes that he or she is trying to do the interview "just right" can recall that families want compassionate clinicians—not perfect ones. The clinician then considers the following practical strategies for giving bad news.

Practical Recommendations for Giving Bad News

A private setting, free of distractions, is required. The clinician arranges for coverage, so beepers or cell phones do not interrupt. All parties should be seated [8]. Both parents should be invited if the discussion is about a child. Any relatives, like grandparents, who parents wish to be present, can be included [8]. Another health professional, such as a nurse, who knows the family well, might be helpful in the process.

Patients express satisfaction when a physician connects with them personally [9]. Although the initial contact may be brief, that personal connection is important. The clinician then checks to see if the patient or family is ready to talk. Experts frequently suggest helping a family prepare to hear bad news by firing off a **warning shot**, such as: *The condition appears to be more serious than I first thought* [10].

It is important for the clinician to be clear and straightforward. He or she will only be able to be clear and effective if the patient's view of the illness is understood first [11].

Clinician	Before we get started, tell me what you know about this type of illness.
Patient	I don't know for sure. I thought it might be a swollen lymph node.

Vagueness and jargon should be avoided. Patients and families generally want to know the diagnosis as soon as the clinician makes the diagnosis [8]. As the clinician shares information, he or she is careful not to rush the process. This is accomplished by letting the patient take the lead. It can be tempting to move quickly to what can be done about the condition, before the patient's feelings of fear and grief have been acknowledged and assimilated [11]. **This temptation should be vigorously avoided or the patient is likely to feel unsupported and falsely reassured.** The clinician pays attention to nonverbal signals from the family, so that he or she does not overwhelm a family with information. Many families need the information given in small chunks. That does not mean they need overly optimistic information. Inaccurate information prevents them from acknowledging and grieving their losses. I have witnessed parents of children holding onto a diagnosis of developmental delay describe their frantic efforts to help their child "catch up," when the child was severely intellectually impaired. An overly negative prognosis does not help families either. One study found that residents adopted a more pessimistic prognosis than faculty when talking with families in the Pediatric Intensive Care Unit [12]. No doubt some residents thought they were protecting the families from experiencing the disappointment of a bad outcome. Although these residents made their prognostic statements with good intentions, families cannot be protected from feeling the pain of loss.

One way for the clinician to monitor his or her pace is to check, and recheck, the family's understanding *throughout* the course of the meeting [8].

Clinician	Let me check out what you have heard me say so far to make sure I have said it clearly.
Patient	You said that the biopsy of the lump in my neck came back as cancer, but you think it was caught early.

Emotional Reaction

Families want and need to first understand **what it all means** in terms of effecting the patient's functioning and quality of life [13]. They may experience difficulty saying that clearly because of their own anxieties. Learning what it all means drives the family's emotional response. It is critical for the clinician to observe nonverbal signals and elicit the family's feelings. The clinician tracks the emotional response of the family from the onset, with comments like: *You look worried* or *I can imagine that it must be overwhelming to hear this news.* Some families protect themselves through a denial of the reality. It feels like it is too much to let in all at once. The clinician expresses empathy for these families by an acceptance of their denial. This state of shock is simply labeled: *I imagine this information seems overwhelming, almost like a shock too hard to comprehend.*

Other families express their sad, broken state, and stay open to receiving empathy from the clinician.

Vann Joines teaches a powerful intervention at the Southeast Institute for Individual, Group, and Family Therapy. He suggests a **feeling** response when a person is grieving and expressing feelings. Questions and statements that invite **thinking** responses often move clients away from heart-to-heart exchanges. Examples of thinking responses might be:

Who will support you as you deal with this news?
It's natural to feel sad when you hear that your child has a chronic lung disease.

Talking about feelings can be educational and important. However, families feel most soothed with heart-to-heart or feeling responses, such as the following: (said softly)

- *It's a big loss.*
- *It's painful.*
- *Put words to your tears.*
- *Silence for 5–30 s.*

I once saw a physician give a feeling response that captures the essence of this response. An elderly woman cried as Dr. Tim Campbell was making his morning rounds. The distraught woman explained that, during the previous night, she had not been allowed to visit with her gravely ill husband of 50 years. Dr. Campbell responded with simple compassion. He hugged the woman. She calmed down and then they talked. I remember the incident because that woman was my mother.

Physicians can allow themselves to **imagine** what the family might be experiencing in order to respond with a feeling or heart-to-heart exchange. Although it can be painful to even imagine what a family is experiencing, a compassionate physician does just that. In a sense, the physician keeps one foot in the patient's experience and one foot out, for he or she cannot really feel the patient's or family's pain. But, the physician can let them know he or she empathizes with what they are experiencing.

Table 19.1 Giving bad news

Do a personal grief inventory, attending to one's own history of loss and grief
Examine for self-talk that might interfere with being fully present to patient
Stay aware of one's feelings in order to manage them and respond empathetically to family
Expert recommendations
Private setting/both parents
Contract (agreement to meet)
Give warning shot
Empathy (*"I imagine…"*)
Give news in chunks
Check family's understanding and emotional response all along the way
Go slowly
Tell them what it *means*
Arrange follow-up

Clinician I imagine it is heartbreaking to hear this type of news about your child.

Patient I do feel like it is too much to bear.

Clinician I wish it were different… (*silence*)

Empathy has a power to soothe when patients and families most need solace. Unfortunately, empirical studies find empathy is too infrequently used by physicians, even those providing care to patients with advanced cancer [14].

The flexible use of these guidelines allows for the unique needs of each family to be compassionately addressed. Studies show that families frequently do not remember much about the session other than the attitude of the physician. Some clinicians record the session and give the tape to the family. Whether or not that is done, all families need a follow-up session. This allows the family to ask questions that have arisen, and for the physician to check in on their emotional state. Any referrals or other specific information likely to be forgotten can be written down for the family (Table 19.1).

Key Points

1. Giving bad news well is an essential part of good medical care.
2. Check that patient understands from the beginning and along the way.
3. Patients need information given in small chunks and with compassion.
4. Tell the patient and family what it means.
5. Respond to the patient's feelings of grief, both verbal and nonverbal. Do not rush to tell the patient what can be done about it.

References

1. Binder J. Pediatric Interviewing: a practical, relationship-based approach. New York, NY: Humana Press; 2010.
2. Fallowfield L. Giving sad and bad news. Lancet. 1993;341:476–8.
3. Remen RN. Kitchen table wisdom. New York, NY: Riverhead Books; 1997.
4. Neimeyer R. Lessons of loss: a guide to coping. Memphis, TN: Center for the Study of Loss and Transition; 2006.
5. Beck JS. Cognitive therapy: basics and beyond. New York, NY: The Guilford Press; 1995.
6. Harris A. Good guys and sweethearts. Trans Anal J III. 1972;1:13–9.
7. Goulding MM. Childhood scenes. In: Lennox CE, editor. Redecision therapy: a brief, action-oriented approach. Northvale, NJ: Jason Aronson; 1997.
8. Girgis A, Sanson-Fisher RW. Breaking bad news: consensus guidelines for medical practitioners. J Clin Oncol. 1995;13:2449–56.
9. Korsch BM, Aley EF. Pediatric interviewing techniques: current pediatric therapy. Sci Am. 1973;3:1–42.
10. Buckman R. How to break bad news: a guide for the health care professional. Baltimore, MD: John Hopkins University Press; 1992.
11. Platt FW, Gordon GH. Field guide to the difficult patient interview. 2nd ed. Philadelphia, PA: Lippincott Williams and Wilkins; 2004.
12. Marcin JP, Pollack MM, Kuntilal MP, Sprague BM, Ruttimann UE. Prognostication and certainty in the pediatric intensive care unit. Pediatrics. 1999;104:868–73.
13. Coulehan JL, Block MR. The medical interview: mastering skills for clinical practice. 5th ed. Philadelphia, PA: FA Davis; 2006.
14. Pollak KI, Arnold RM, Jeffreys AS, Alexander SC, Olsen MK, Abernethy AP, et al. Oncologist communication about emotions during visits with patients with advanced cancer. J Clin Oncol. 2007;25:5748–52.

Chapter 20
Challenging Interviews

Role Play

Master the following prerequisite skills before role-playing challenging interviews: ***contracting, open-ended inquiry***, *eliciting and responding to feelings, uncovering patient's **theory of illness**,* and *taking a family approach.*

Since strong negative affective reactions by patients are integral to challenging interview role plays, it is useful to have trained actors and actresses play the part of patients.

Role Play #1:   A 26-year-old woman with a chief complaint of recurrent abdominal pain. Physical exam reveals cutting on her wrists and forearms. She acknowledges she has been cutting, but refuses a referral for mental health counseling.

Objectives

1. Maintain a collaborative stance with the patient.
2. Develop a contract for the next step.

Trainee	I would like to talk to you about the cuts on your wrists and arms.
Patient	Okay.
Trainee	Tell me about them.
Patient	When I get real upset, I cut myself. I haven't done it in a week.
Trainee	So you are trying to stop?
Patient	I would like to stop.
Trainee	Are you trying to hurt yourself when you do it?

(continued)

J. Binder, *Primary Care Interviewing: Learning Through Role Play*,
DOI 10.1007/978-1-4614-7224-7_20, © Springer Science+Business Media New York 2013

Patient	I just get so upset and feel so bad. I don't know what else to do.
Trainee	Do you ever wish you were dead?
Patient	Fleeting thoughts. I do not want to die.
Trainee	Have you ever cut yourself hoping you would die?
Patient	Never.
Trainee	A minute ago you said you would like to stop cutting. I would like to refer you to somebody who specializes in helping people learn ways of managing their feelings in a safe way.
Patient	I don't think that is necessary.
Trainee	Would you tell me more about not wanting to see a counselor.
Patient	I've gone before when I was a teenager. It was a waste of time.
Trainee	I'm sorry to hear that you had a bad experience. There are many different ways of counseling. I know someone who has helped a number of people with difficulties similar to yours learn how to regulate their emotions.
Patient	I'm sure that may be true. I still don't want to go.
Trainee	The problem is that I am not an expert in this area and it is important for you to see a specialist.
Patient	*(turns head and body away from the interviewer)*

Feedback

Faculty	Okay, let's stop here. *(To trainee)* Tell me what you are experiencing.
Trainee	I'm frustrated. She's self-destructive and, in addition, won't agree to see a specialist who could help her.
Faculty	I can appreciate why you are frustrated. It is a difficult situation. Anything else you are experiencing?
Trainee	I feel somewhat anxious. I don't feel qualified to handle a patient like her—who is cutting herself.
Faculty	What are you saying to yourself, specifically?
Trainee	What happens if she starts cutting more and really hurts herself, perhaps putting herself at risk of dying? I don't want to take responsibility for that.
Faculty	So you imagine feeling helpless and responsible for her as her condition worsens? Is there any anger with all this?
Trainee	Sure. She is being so uncooperative.
Faculty	I see why you are trying so hard to get her to go to a specialist. The only problem is that she is not willing to go. Would you be open to another way of looking at the situation? It might help you with your anxiety.

(continued)

Trainee	What do you mean?
Faculty	I think you would feel less anxious if you developed a true partnership. The first step is recognizing that you have hit a bump in the road—that this is a challenging interview. If you step back for a second, how would you diagnose the interaction?
Trainee	We have a difference of opinion about a mental health referral.
Faculty	What do you think would be a useful next step?
Trainee	I know it is important with disagreements to first listen to the patient's perspective and find common ground.
Faculty	Terrific. So, what you might consider is to invite the patient to tell you her perspective and listen carefully. You will need to make sure that she knows you have really heard her. A good way to accomplish that is to carefully summarize the details of her perspective. It would be critical to summarize her view in a concerned manner, emphasize points of agreement, and don't rush the process.
Trainee	I think I was trying to convince her before really listening to her story.
Faculty	Wonderful awareness! Are you ready to replay it? This time, will you invite her to talk openly before asking for specifics?
Trainee	Yes.

Replay

Trainee	I would like to go back for a second. I don't think I asked you about your view of the situation. Would you tell me your perspective?
Patient	What do you mean?
Trainee	I have not heard what you think. You said you do not think a referral is necessary. Would you tell me more?
Patient	Well, it's a little hard to talk about. I feel ashamed.
Trainee	Say more.
Patient	I started scratching my wrists in eighth grade. My best friend was doing it. It has become a habit.
Trainee	Tell me more.
Patient	Whenever I feel bad, I cut myself without even thinking about it.
Trainee	So you have been scratching or cutting since eighth grade. It has become somewhat of a habit whenever you feel very bad. You experience shame, and have a hard time talking about it. I appreciate your courage in talking about it today.

(continued)

Patient	Thanks.
Trainee	When you say you cut because you feel bad, what do you mean?
Patient	Sometimes I criticize myself if I have a problem in a relationship. I withdraw and feel bad. The only relief I can get is to cut myself. It helps temporarily.
Trainee	Let me see if I am hearing you correctly… You started cutting years ago. You do it to give yourself some temporary relief from emotional pain. You don't see other options for relieving the pain, especially in relationships. It has become a habit. You feel shame about it.
Patient	That's it.
Trainee	What, if anything, would you like to do about it?
Patient	I don't know. I know I don't want to talk to a counselor. I think that would make me feel worse.
Trainee	If you think seeing a counselor would make you feel worse, no wonder you don't want to go. Would it be okay if I tell you one concern I have?
Patient	Okay.
Trainee	I am concerned that by eliminating the possibility of a referral to a specialist, you are missing out on the possibility of learning other ways of dealing with painful feelings that would work better than cutting.
Patient	Maybe, but I'm not ready to find out.
Trainee	I hear you. Let's talk about ways we could work together. We both want to relieve your emotional pain.

Feedback

Faculty	Okay, let's stop there. (*To trainee*) Tell me what you like about your interview.
Trainee	I felt much better the second time. I felt calm and in control. I thought I listened well.
Patient	I agree. I thought you were really interested in my view. You seemed concerned. I especially liked the way you said we would work together to relieve my emotional pain.
Faculty	I wrote down so many positives. You started off by saying, "I would like to go back." A wonderful thing about interviews is the ability to go back and redo something when it hasn't gone well. You repeatedly used gentle commands to open up the patient. You gave her space to talk. You summarized, using her words and giving details, letting her know you really understood her view. You had a concerned tone of voice. You identified a common goal: to relieve emotional pain.

(continued)

> You do have options for working together: assess for depression, help her with problem solving, and possibly invite family members in for a family session. Great job!

Role Play #2: A 61-year-old man is seeing his primary care physician for a sinus infection. During a checkup six months ago, he had lab work done. His PSA was 12. The clinician realizes he never discussed the results with the patient.

Objectives

1. Acknowledge a medical mistake
2. Elicit and respond to the patient's emotions at a feeling level (heart-to-heart exchange)

Trainee	I would like to talk to you about something that is difficult.
Patient	Yes?
Trainee	One of the tests I ordered when you were here six months ago was for Prostate Specific Antigen or PSA for short. This is a test for a protein that comes from the prostate. When it is high, an abnormality in the prostate is likely. Your result was 12, which is very high. The result was placed in your chart before I reviewed it. I never contacted you. I am very sorry.
Patient	What does a high result mean?
Trainee	It suggests an abnormality in the prostate.
Patient	What kind of abnormality?
Trainee	Any number of conditions could cause this. I would like to repeat the test first, to see if it is accurate. If it is, you will need to see a urologist.
Patient	What kind of abnormalities are you talking about?
Trainee	(*to faculty*) Do I need to be specific before I repeat the test?

Feedback

Faculty	Tell me what you think.
Trainee	I think so. It's just hard to say the words aloud to him—that he may have cancer that has progressed without treatment for 6 months because of my mistake.

(continued)

Faculty	It sure is. What are you saying to yourself about this mistake?
Trainee	'He is going to be so angry.' 'He probably will sue.' 'I let him down.' 'What kind of doctor am I?' Stuff like that.
Faculty	It is hard to talk to him when you are thinking all these thoughts. I have an idea. Are you willing to do an experiment?
Trainee	What is it?
Faculty	Let's enlist a group member to whisper those thoughts in your ear as you talk to the patient. We will externalize what you are doing internally.
Trainee	I'm willing to try it out.
Faculty	Who would like to play the role of the doctor's thoughts?
Group Member	I will.
Faculty	Okay, stand over there and whisper his thoughts as he talks to the patient.

Replay

Patient	What kind of abnormalities can cause this?
Trainee	Well a number of conditions can cause this.
Group Member	(*whispering in trainee's ear*) He is really going to be pissed.
Trainee	One of the conditions is . . . .
Group Member	(*whispering in trainee's ear*) You really screwed up. What kind of doctor are you?
Trainee	Possible causes include... (*stops and laughs*) I can't talk when someone is whispering in my ear.
Faculty	What are you experiencing?
Trainee	I am stuck in my own thoughts and not really listening to the patient.
Faculty	Nice awareness. Are you ready to replay this interview and leave the internal self-critical statements out of the conversation? If you notice them reappear, you might set them aside. It would be natural to feel remorse about this situation. Those feelings are best dealt with by talking with others, such as a peer consultation group.
Trainee	I'm ready.

Replay

Patient	What kinds of abnormalities can this cause?
Trainee	A number of different problems with the prostate, including cancer.
Patient	Cancer?
Trainee	I imagine it is incredibly hard to hear this.
Patient	You can't imagine, doctor! This is my life, and it's your fault.
Trainee	I want you to know how sorry I am.
Patient	I thought I was coming in for a sinus infection and you are telling me I might have cancer and that you didn't tell me for 6 months.
Trainee	No wonder you are so angry with me.
Patient	It is just so hard to believe.
Trainee	(*listens silently*)
Patient	It's very upsetting.
Trainee	(*listens silently*)
Patient	What do I need to do now?
Trainee	The first thing is to repeat the test.
Patient	Then what?
Trainee	I would like to see you back later this week, discuss the results of the repeat test and decide together what would be the next step. Are you willing to return?
Patient	I will return later this week. I'm not sure about after that.
Trainee	Of course.

Feedback

Faculty	Let's stop here. (*to trainee*) What did you experience with this interview?
Trainee	Although it was difficult, I thought I stayed in contact with him and his feelings. I didn't try to bypass his feelings.
Faculty	I agree. I thought you did a terrific job of not getting defensive and of supporting his feelings. It was a beautiful example of a heart-to-heart exchange.

Obstacles to Teaching Challenging Interviews

1. Interviewer believes that challenging interviews are solely the result of patient characteristics.
2. Interviewer believes that the skills needed to handle a challenging interview are for experts only.
3. Interviewer is unaware of his or her own emotional reactions to challenging patients.

Strategies

1. Encourage a trainee to experience the patient role, so he or she can experience the impact of different styles of interviewing.
2. Demonstrate how good basic interviewing skills can help manage many challenging interviews.
3. Teach trainees about the connection between family-of-origin issues and interacting with patients in the present.

Challenging Interviews

Examples of challenging interviews are scattered through this book: suicidal patients, shutdown adolescents, somatically fixated patients, patients receiving bad news, disruptive families, etc. In this chapter, an approach to challenging patients, based on the outline put forward by Maysel Kemp White and Vaughn Keller, is reviewed. Their approach grew directly out of numerous physician–patient communication workshops given at the Bayer Institute for Healthcare Communications [1]. Two types of clinical situations, which overlap with the above categories, were identified as particularly difficult: handling strong negative emotional reactions of patients and dealing with self-destructive behavior of patients—such as smoking and gluttony—for which they didn't seem to be taking responsibility [2]. The common theme in these two types of clinical encounters was the strong negative affect experienced by many clinicians. The emotional reactions appeared to be "hot button" issues.

If clinicians do not recognize these emotional hot spots, the interview will spiral downward. Challenging interviews can be recognized by staying self-aware (something feels uncomfortable) and paying attention to the process of the interview. Interruptions and repetitions suggest the interview is in trouble [1]. Once a challenging interview is recognized, a critical task of the clinician is to control and manage his or her own negative feelings. Self-reflection, peer group consultation, and psychotherapy can support that capacity [3]. An unaware clinician is likely to respond with defensiveness and attempt to prove that he or she is right [4]. Only after negative affect is controlled can the interviewer effectively utilize other techniques to assess and repair the disruption to the relationship. The following tools, discussed in the previous chapters (2, 3, 5, 6, and 13), allow the clinician to organize a logical approach to challenging interviews: contracting, empathizing, understanding the meaning of the problem, and involving the family [1].

Contract

Once the clinician recognizes a disruption to the relationship, and before efforts to repair that disruption are made, a new contract must be established. The clinician asks the patient if he or she is willing to deal with the disruption to the relationship. An example might be [5]:

| Clinician | I sense you are unhappy about what I just said (or did). If that is true, would you be willing to talk about it? |
| Patient | I have a problem with your handling of the situation. |

Contracting provides the boundaries needed for emotional safety. A patient might not be ready to discuss a relationship problem. If the patient is willing to discuss the problem, it is done respectfully. Disruptive behavior is rare, but clear limits must be firmly maintained when it is experienced.

Patient	(*loud voice*) What kind of stupid doctor are you?
Clinician	I hear that you are really angry with me. It is hard for me to listen to you when you raise your voice so loudly, but I do want to hear you. I am going to leave the office for a few minutes. When I return, I would like to talk this out with you. Are you agreeable?
Comment	*If the clinician felt in any danger, supervisory staff should be alerted.*

Empathic Communication

Empathy is the cornerstone of an effective response to many difficult interviews. Empathic communication, especially when vulnerable feelings of fear, sadness, and loss are shared, brings the patient and clinician together after they have experienced a disruption in their relationship [2]. Serious disruptions can take repeated interactions of empathy and soothing over time. Although empathy is a simple concept to comprehend, it is not so simple to accomplish when the patient and clinician have intense feelings that block effective communication.

A clinician experiencing anxiety, frustration, or any number of other emotions might distract the conversation away from the patient's feelings in order to avoid an awkward moment [6], as in the following inquiry:

| Patient | I feel exhausted from the medicine you started me on for my nerves. I can't even get small tasks finished. I feel worthless. |
| Clinician | You must be extra sensitive to this kind of medication. Have you noticed that with other medicines? |

Some clinicians, like the above clinician, are unaware of how their own feelings influence clinical interactions. Experienced teachers recommend trainees stop and reflect a moment whenever they sense a patient is experiencing a strong feeling [2]. The trainee follows up with questioning until the patient's feelings can be labeled and acknowledged [2]. One of the important advantages of performing role plays, and repeatedly observing peers' role play, is the increased awareness trainees develop recognizing and naming feelings.

Patients also place barriers in the way of empathic communication. Platt and Keller identified two situations in which patients block empathy [2]. Patients who are angry about a clinician's error will require an apology before they are likely to accept empathic statements. Other patients view empathy as pity or an intrusion into their personal space. A respectful approach is to label the defense and not persist: *I get a sense that you are the type of person who likes to keep a stiff upper lip.*

Most patients will accept and respond to genuine empathy. It is crucial for the clinician to fully listen to the patient before stating his or her view, if different from the patient's [7]. The clinician lets the patient know he or she has listened by carefully summarizing all the details and feelings communicated by the patient. The clinician continues to summarize until the patient indicates the clinician understands correctly [8] (see Role Play #1 at the beginning of this chapter).

Meaning of Illness or Problem

The functional and symbolic meaning the patient attributes to the problem will drive the emotional reaction [9]. This may or may not be readily apparent. Direct questioning is typically all that is required, perhaps with a little persistence.

Patient	I can't do much of anything. I feel exhausted just cooking a meal.
Clinician	So, you have really experienced a major loss of being able to do tasks.
Patient	I have.
Clinician	What do you see as the cause of this?
Patient	I'm not sure.
Clinician	If you had to guess, what would you say?
Patient	To tell you the truth, I think I must have some sickness. I know you say I'm depressed, but I don't think that is causing me to feel so bad.

Include Family

As the most powerful social system that influences patients, it can be helpful to include their families [10]. Family members can be invited to a visit or the clinician can offer to make a home visit. The clinician can "think family," even with individual patients, by asking family-related questions (e.g., *Who in the family would be helpful in dealing with the problem?*) [11]. Family members may bring a different perspective and new solutions.

Clinician	Mrs. James, if I am hearing you right, you are totally exhausted and can't get your daily tasks done. You are frustrated with me because you don't believe that it is due to depression. You are concerned we may be missing a serious, underlying illness. Is that it?
Patient	Yes.
Clinician	I often find it helpful to include other family members when I get stuck. They can bring a fresh perspective. Would it be okay if we invite your husband to your next visit?
Patient	I'm not sure what good that would do, but if you think it might help, I'm sure he would come.
Clinician	You and I have different views about the cause of your symptoms. I have diagnosed a depression. You are concerned that I might be missing something. You don't think inviting your husband to a visit will help, but you are willing. I do think it might help.
Patient	Okay.

Key Points

1. A challenging interview can be recognized subjectively (something is wrong) and objectively (interruptions, repetitions, etc.).
2. It is critical for the interviewer to be aware of and manage his or her own feelings and to not personalize the situation.
3. A new contract to deal with the relationship rupture is the first step.
4. It is also important to understand the meaning of an illness or problem to the patient.
5. Empathize with the patient's feelings, particularly vulnerable feelings of fear, sadness, and loss.
6. Let the patient know you really understand his or her perspective by carefully summarizing the details of their perspective before expressing your concerns.

References

1. White MK, Keller VF. Difficult clinician-patient relationships. J Clin Outcomes Manag. 1998;5:32–6.
2. Platt FW, Keller VF. Empathic communication: a teachable and learnable skill. J Gen Intern Med. 1994;9:222–6.
3. Novack DH, Suchman AL, Clark W, Epstein RM, Najberg E, Kaplan C. Calibrating the physician: personal awareness and effective patient care. Working Group on Promoting Personal Awareness, American Academy on Physician and Patient. JAMA. 1997;278:502–9.
4. McDaniel SH, Campbell TC, Hepworth J, Lorenz A. Family-oriented primary care. 2nd ed. New York, NY: Springer; 2005.
5. Carson CA. Nonverbal communication. In: Cole SA, Bird J, editors. The medical interview: the three-function approach. 2nd ed. Philadelphia, PA: Mosby; 2006.
6. Epstein RM, Morse DS, Frankel RM, Frarey L, Anderson K, Beckman HB. Awkward moments in patient-physician communication about HIV risk. Ann Intern Med. 1998;128:435–42.
7. Platt FW, Gordon GH. Field guide to the difficult patient interview. 2nd ed. Philadelphia, PA: Lippincott Williams and Wilkins; 2004.
8. Platt FW, Prose NS. Training the trainers: a seminar for teachers of doctor-patient communication. Workshop presented at Duke University Medical Center, Durham, NC, May 4, 2010.
9. Martin AR. Exploring patient beliefs: steps to enhancing physician-patient interaction. Arch Intern Med. 1983;143:1773–5.
10. Campbell TL. The effectiveness of family interventions in the treatment of physical illness. J Marital Fam Ther. 2003;29:263–81.
11. Cole-Kelly K, Seaburn D. Five areas of questioning to promote a family-oriented approach in primary care. Fam Syst Health. 1999;17:340–8.

Appendix A

Five Steps to an Efficient Primary Care Visit

1. Agree to a **clear contract** for what will be dealt with during the visit. Consider the priority of the symptoms and time available when negotiating the agenda. Be realistic. Keep in mind situations that may require extra time, such as many psychosocial problems. The contract demarcates the content of subsequent phases of the interview.
2. Once the opening phase of the interview has been completed, get the patient on track: *I would like to hear about your glucose monitoring and how you have managed low and high readings over the last month.*
3. Stay in one region until it is finished, other than to respond to a patient's feelings or immediate needs. Use an open-ended to closed-ended questioning technique (funneling) to expand the region. Cover any lists, such as the review of systems, by using the gentle command: *Stop me if you have had any of the following...* (Platt, August, 2012).
4. Guide the interview between and within regions with transition statements (see Chap. 7). Use progressive structuring if the patient wanders.
5. From the start, plan to leave adequate time to discuss your assessment and develop a treatment plan together. Complete your evaluation before initiating that discussion. Do not rush; efficient interviews require a strongly engaged patient.

Note: Experience helps clinicians learn to recognize patterns, know when it is safe to do abbreviated scanning, and what questions discriminate between conditions—all of which help them to be more efficient.

J. Binder, *Primary Care Interviewing: Learning Through Role Play*,   255
DOI 10.1007/978-1-4614-7224-7, © Springer Science+Business Media New York 2013

Appendix B

Suggested Readings

1. Platt F, Gordon G. Field guide to the difficult patient interview. Philadelphia, PA: Lippincott Williams & Wilkins; 2004.
2. Fortin A, Dwamena F, Frankel R, Smith R. Smith's patient-centered interviewing: an evidence-based method. 3rd ed. New York, NY: McGraw-Hill; 2012.
3. McDaniel S, Campbell T, Hepworth J, Lorenz A. Family-oriented primary care. 2nd ed. New York, NY: Springer; 2005.
4. Rollnick S, Miller W, Butler C. Motivational interview in health care: helping patients change behavior. New York, NY: Guilford Press; 2008.
5. Shea S. Improving medication adherence: how to talk with patients about their medications. Philadelphia, PA: Lippincott, Williams & Wilkins; 2006.
6. Novack D, Clark W, Daetwyler C, Saizon R, editors. Doc.com: an interactive learning resource for healthcare communication (c). http://webcompus.drexel/med-edu/doc.com/

J. Binder, *Primary Care Interviewing: Learning Through Role Play*,
DOI 10.1007/978-1-4614-7224-7, © Springer Science+Business Media New York 2013

Glossary of Interviewing Terms

Affirmation Any verbal or nonverbal behavior that focuses on and shows appreciation for the positive actions or intentions of another person.

Attending The state of being fully present to the nonverbal and verbal communications of another person.

Behavioral incident Specific historical details of a behavior or symptom are asked about in a chronological fashion to obtain valid data and not opinion.

Cannon questions Successive questions asked before the interviewee has a chance to answer the first one, leaving the interviewee unclear about which question to answer.

Circular questioning The interviewer asks questions that are based on the thoughts, feelings, and behaviors just expressed by another member of the family. For example, "Tell me what you experience, Mrs. Jones, when your husband says he feels trapped by his diabetes." The interviewer can subsequently return to the original family member to complete the circle.

Closing the window An interviewing technique for concluding an excursion into an emotional or personal area and returning to the original topic.

Contact The level of connection that the interviewer has to the experience of the patient. It can also refer to the extent that the interviewer is in touch with his or her own thoughts and feelings.

Continuers Brief nonverbal or verbal (e.g., uh-huh) responses of the interviewer that facilitate the conversation.

Contract An agreement between two autonomous people to a well-defined course of action.

Echoing The act of repeating back to the patient part, or all, of what the patient just said as a way of encouraging the patient to say more about that part of the communication.

Emphatic summary Stating back to the patient what the clinician has so far heard the patient say in terms of medical data, thoughts, feelings, and values. A summary has three parts: a stem ("Let me see if I have this right …"), the summary itself, and a brief period of silence at the conclusion.

J. Binder, *Primary Care Interviewing: Learning Through Role Play*,
DOI 10.1007/978-1-4614-7224-7, © Springer Science+Business Media New York 2013

Enactment A term from family therapy: two members of a family or group interact in front of the interviewer. The interviewer assigns a task and then observes the interactions.

Engagement The connection between interviewer and interviewee that supports the interviewee feeling safe and becoming activated to talk.

Externalize A gestalt technique, which can be designed to help an interviewer to develop the self-awareness that he or she is not listening to what the patient is saying. The trainee's thoughts, usually self-critical, are whispered into the ear of that trainee (by another group member) as he or she tries to talk with a patient.

Facilitate Brief verbal and nonverbal cues from the interviewer, inviting the patient to continue the conversation (e.g., "uh-huh").

Feeling response A nonverbal or verbal reaction or statement of the interviewer that invites a heart-to-heart (emotional) exchange with a patient.

Focused (questioning) Interviewer inquiry that invites the patient to provide more details and a deeper understanding of a topic.

Gates Also called ties, these are transition statements joining two different areas of the history.

> **Implied** Moving to a new topic that is generally related to the previous topic. The transition is *implied* by the similarity of the subject matter.

> **Introduced** The interviewer moves to a new topic by simply stating he or she is making a transition (e.g., "I would now like to ask about your past medical history").

> **Referred** The interviewer moves to a new topic by going back to an earlier statement made by the interviewee.

Gentle assumption The interviewer asks a question assuming the interviewee has a certain thought or is performing a certain behavior. This technique can increase validity. It should not be used when asking about a history of abuse, since this could lead to false reporting.

Gentle command An open-ended request that often has no question mark attached to it and starts with:

Tell me …

Describe …

Say something about …

A gentle or caring voice is used.

Heart-to-heart exchange The interviewer and patient connect at a feeling level.

Hidden agenda An unstated worry of a parent present in many childhood illness visits. Of course, calling it "hidden" is a bit of a misnomer. It is only hidden until asked about with inquires such as "What else can you tell me?" or "What concerns you the most?" Such questions are part of a good interviewer's armamentarium and do not require blaming the patient for hiding something.

Listening "Being quiet and paying attention to the person who's talking" (Platt and Gordon, p.15).

Nonverbal communication Behavioral signals sent by the interviewer or patient that communicate messages that are typically out of the subject's awareness.

The categories of nonverbal signals are kinesics, proxemics, paralanguage, and autonomic output (see Chap. 3).

Normalization A technique to decrease defensiveness and increase accuracy by acknowledging the universality of feelings or some other human experience. This often decreases the interviewee's sense of shame and isolation.

Open-ended Inquiries that are not easily answered in one or two words.

Personalize The process of emotionally reacting on the basis of early childhood *decisions* about self and other people rather than the here-and-now reality.

Personal story Learning about the person in the patient, who and what are important in the patient's life.

Pivot point A choice an interviewer has to make between moving with the patient in a new direction and referring back to the previous topic.

Progressive structuring An interviewing approach to focusing wandering patients in which the intensity of the interventions is gradually increased.

Rapport See Engagement.

Region The interview stays on a topic for several sentences or more.

Restate The patient tells the clinician what he heard the clinician say. It is a way to check, recall, and understand. Also called Echoing Back and Short Summary.

Reverse role play A trainee role-plays the patient while the teacher demonstrates an interviewing technique.

Role play A technique in which a clinician–patient interview situation is created with a trainee taking on the role of the clinician. Volunteers or trained actors/actresses play the roles of patients or family. Trainees and faculty negotiate objectives for the exercise before the start of the interaction.

Safety An environment that is nurturing, accepting, and nonjudgmental of interviewee's experience. This encourages an interviewee to talk, free from the scare that he or she will be judged critically.

Self-awareness Novack et al. define self-awareness as the process of developing in the present moment "insights into how one's life experiences and emotional makeup affect one's interactions with patients, families, and other professionals."

Setting the stage The interviewer inquires about non-sensitive topics before asking about sensitive issues, in order to give the patient time to feel comfortable with the interviewer.

Theory of illness The patient's ideas about the cause and symbolic meaning of his or her symptoms.

Third-person technique A normalization technique developed by Michael Rothenberg. The interviewer bypasses interviewee defensiveness by saying, "Lots of people in this situation …." He or she then states what lots of people might feel or think in that situation. This is followed by asking the patient if that makes sense to him or her. Finally, is it true for the patient?

Tracking The interviewer attends to the feelings and experience of the interviewee by asking questions or making comments that flow directly from the statements of the interviewee.

Transition See Gates.

Validity tools Interviewing techniques that increase the likelihood of receiving accurate information.

Warning shot A brief statement made before giving bad news so patient and family can prepare themselves.

Weave Integrating an open-ended inquiry into an area of more focused questioning.

Index

A

AACAP. *See* American Academy of Child &
Adolescent Psychiatry (AACAP)
Accuracy
high control interview and, 88
ignoring psychosocial data, 88
insufficient inquiry, 88
lack of details, 1, 90
not summarizing, 89
Across the life span, 119–132
Adolescents
building a relationship, 124
contracting with, 29, 127, 129, 132, 215, 217
interviewing, 5, 29, 123, 124, 126, 128,
129, 214, 216, 250
Adolescent sexual history
confidentiality and, 215
contracting, 215
normalization, 216–217
set the stage, 215–216
Affirmations
empirical support, 45–46
personal responsibility, 47
practical points, 46–48
Alcohol use disorders
abuse and dependence, 225, 226, 229
assessment, 225–227, 229
CAGE, 225, 226
clinician frustration, 225
family support, 224, 225, 228, 229
motivational interviewing, 224–227
screen, 224, 225
Ambivalence, 199, 224, 228
American Academy of Child & Adolescent
Psychiatry (AACAP), 200
Anchor points, 91

Anger, 7, 52, 53, 56, 57, 199, 233–235, 244
Anxious patient/family
slower pace, 125

B

Barriers to role play
anxiety, 2
beliefs about role play, 2
Bayer Institute for Healthcare
Communications, 250
Behavioral incidents, 91, 93, 94, 149, 163,
189, 257
Being with patients, 240
Benefits of role play
assessment of trainees, 1
broad applicability, 1
evidence-based, 1
Berne, E., 27
Betancourt, J.R., 142
Biopsychosocial approach
in primary care, 17, 143
Brief interventions with alcohol use disorders
elicit-provide-elicit, 227
give specific recommendations, 229
roll with resistance, 228
support change, 228–229

C

CAGE, 225–226
Carter, B., 141
Challenging interviews
examples of, 29, 249, 250
negative clinician affect, 243, 250
recognizing emotional hot spots, 250

Circular questioning, 149, 163, 186, 257
Clarification of symptoms, 90, 101, 113
Class divided, 139, 159
Clever hunch, 100
Closed-ended questions
    series of, 35, 99, 106
Closing phase of interview
    give and take, 112, 114, 117
    importance, 113
    time needed, 113
Closing the window, 60, 78, 158, 257
Cognitive deficit
    dementia, delirium, 89
    nonverbal empathy and, 90
Collaborative Family Health Care Model,
    174–178
Common language
    join, 159
Computers, 29, 75
Concerns
    vs. worry, 55, 258
Confrontation, 36, 39, 43, 199, 224
Consultation groups, 248
Contact
    before contract, 27, 28, 30
Context for hpi
    clinical, 107
Contracting
    definition, 25
    expectations, 5, 25–27, 35, 76
    positively framed, 28
    psychosocial issues, 25, 27, 28
    renegotiable, 25, 28, 30, 160
    specific, clear, 2, 24–26, 76, 160
Conversational style
    gentle commands, 106
    summarize, 107
    weave, 106
Cultural humility
    patient-centered interviewing, 142

D
Deficit model
    healthcare, 45
Denial of the specific, 91, 92, 202, 226
Depression, 17, 45, 78, 79, 91, 92, 127,
    128, 131, 135, 137, 141,
    167–171, 173, 174, 181, 184,
    189, 192, 193, 195–197, 199,
    200, 204, 205, 215, 226, 247,
    252, 253
Diagnostic acumen
    self-awareness, 9

Differential diagnosis
    mental health, 173, 174
    primary care, 17, 173, 174
Doctor, The, 5, 15, 16, 24, 25, 27, 29, 32, 47,
    55, 76, 79, 95–97, 102, 103, 114,
    116, 120, 125, 127, 129, 143, 144,
    150, 160, 165, 172, 182, 215, 237,
    248, 249, 251

E
Elicit-provide-elicit (EPE) structure, 113, 222
Emotional literacy, 56–57
Emotions
    bad news, 8, 235–237, 239–240, 250
    clues, 54, 55
    deepen, 52, 53, 58–59
    direct inquiry, 55, 59
    indirect inquiry, 55, 56
    interpersonal functions, 57
Empathic summaries
    silence after, 38, 58, 95, 103, 257
    stem, 38, 58, 257
Enactment, 149, 163, 164, 258
EPE structure. *See* Elicit-provide-elicit
    (EPE) structure
Evaluate family problems
    circular questioning, 149, 163, 186, 257
    enactment, 149, 163, 164, 258
    specific example, 139, 144, 160
Explanatory model
    uncovering mistaken beliefs, 63, 66–69
Explanatory, social risk, fears, therapeutic
    contracting (ESFT) model, 142

F
Family
    conference, 146, 158, 166, 186
    definition, 104, 137, 139
    influence on health, 137, 138, 142, 143
    involvement, 131, 132, 137, 143–144, 160,
        161, 164, 174, 184, 195, 205
    level of functioning, 138–139
    process, 3, 7, 80, 114, 138, 140, 147, 159,
        160, 163, 164, 237, 238, 250, 259
    structure/systems, 29, 56, 72, 73, 75, 78,
        80, 81, 137–139, 141, 158, 166,
        170, 171, 176, 177, 196, 204
    therapy, 8, 138, 139, 165, 177, 239, 258
    through time, 138, 141
    visits, 80, 144–147, 166
Family interview
    structure of, 29, 81, 154, 158, 166

Family process
  belief about okayness, 140
  differentiation, 140
  mood, 141
  stroking pattern, 140–141
Family through time
  life cycle stages, 141
Family visits
  family conference, 146, 166
  routine, 144–146, 166
  think family, 146–147
Fear
  intense, 59–60, 198, 251
Feedback
  affirmations, 6, 14, 22, 32, 42–45, 64,
      72, 84, 120, 122, 150, 153, 190,
      196, 208, 221
  options, 6, 7, 14, 22, 23, 32, 42, 44, 50,
      65, 72, 85, 86, 121, 122, 151,
      153, 156, 169, 190, 196, 209,
      221, 234, 247
  taking notes, 6
Feelings
  elicit, 9, 27, 36, 50–61, 91, 109, 119, 135,
      143, 149, 155, 171, 189, 207, 224,
      233, 239, 243, 247
  empathic summary, 4, 38, 57, 58, 60, 61,
      156, 182, 185, 233
  reflection, 7, 39, 57, 58, 171, 221,
      237, 252
Five basic questions
  closing phase, 113, 114, 117
Flipchart, 4
Focused questions
  associated symptoms, 102, 105
  chronology, 102–104, 173
  position, 102–104
  quality, 102–105
  quantity, 102–105
  setting, 102, 104, 106
  transforming factors, 102, 104

G
Genogram, 141
Gentle assumption, 91, 92, 226, 258
Gentle commands, 4, 13, 31, 32, 38, 41, 49,
      50, 63, 71, 83, 96, 102, 103, 106,
      154, 246, 255, 258
Geriatrics
  clinician's beliefs, 124, 130, 131
  comprehensive assessment, 130, 131
  family involvement, 124, 130
  hearing loss, 131, 132
  impaired functioning, 131

Giving bad news
  avoid vagueness, 238
  check understanding, 233, 238, 240
  chunk information, 234, 238, 240
  contracting, 240
  interfering beliefs, 240
  meaning to patient/family, 237–240, 260
  practical recommendations, 237–238
  private setting, 237, 240
  slow pace, 234
  support feelings, 236
  warning shot, 238, 240, 260
Gottman, J., 45
Group
  discuss problematic reactions, 8
Guiding the interview, 16, 130

H
Hearing loss, 131, 132, 184, 207
Heart-to-heart, 60, 239, 247, 249, 258
Highly distressed families
  problem solving and, 138
History of present illness
  clinical approach, 1
  preliminary work, 100–101
HIV. See Human immunodeficiency virus (HIV)
Human immunodeficiency virus (HIV),
      60, 212–214

I
Identify mental health disorders
  core interviewing skills, 171–173
  screen, 171
  surveillance, 171
Imagine
  empathy and, 4, 58, 65, 87, 239, 240
Incongruence
  verbal and nonverbal, 39, 54
Integration
  physical and emotional, 17, 184
Interview
  under control, 9, 160
  over control, 8, 56
  patient perception, 73
  practice skills, 1, 4, 7, 10, 73, 135, 219
  structured, 16, 29, 53, 56, 71, 73–78, 80,
      81, 124, 158, 169–171, 173, 178,
      211, 214, 222, 224, 255, 259
  unstructured, 73
Interviewing skills (core)
  engagement, 124, 172
  partnership, 124, 170–172
  structuring, 71, 170–173

J
Joy, 56, 57

K
Kadis, L.B., 137
Keller, V.F., 229, 250, 252
Kemp-White, M., 229, 250
Kinesics, 36, 37, 259
Kleinman, A., 66

L
Lead
  nonverbal, 37, 238
Leadership
  family session, 160
Level of clinician involvement with
    families, 143
Level of functioning
  higher functioning families, 139
  highly distressed families, 138, 139
Listening, 3, 13, 14, 21, 31, 32, 35–37, 39, 41,
    42, 49, 58, 63, 71–73, 79, 83, 89,
    90, 95, 97, 109, 124, 138, 139, 149,
    153, 158–160, 162, 164, 169, 171,
    181, 183, 185, 196, 233, 236, 237,
    245, 246, 248, 249, 251, 252, 258

M
Macrotraining, 135, 149, 154, 201
Match
  nonverbal, 37, 39, 159
McClendon, R., 137
McGoldrick, M., 141
Meaning of illness, 252
Means restriction counseling, 197, 204, 205
Mental assessment
  core interviewing skills for, 167, 170–173
Mental health
  primary care and, 170, 171, 173–178,
    201, 204
Mental health conditions
  under diagnosed and untreated, 170
Mental health referrals, 166, 176–177,
    199, 245
Mini contracts
  ask permission, 28
Minuchin, S., 139
Misperceptions about illness
  uncover, 113
Mortality in primary care
  secondary to lifestyle, 224

Motivational interviewing
  alcohol use disorders, 224–229
  elicit-provide-elicit, 222, 227, 229, 230
  principles, 224, 226
  roll with resistance, 222, 223, 228
  support change, 224, 228–229

N
National Heart, Lung, and Blood Institute, 138
Negotiate
  mutually acceptable diagnosis, 185–186
Nonverbal communication
  empathy, 36, 90
  kinesics, 36, 37, 259
  paralanguage, 36, 37, 259
  proxemics, 36, 259
Normalization, 36, 39, 56–58, 85, 86, 91–92,
    94, 126, 143, 177, 196, 200–201,
    207, 208, 216–217, 225, 259

O
Objectives of role play, 3, 4, 6, 8, 10, 51–52,
    99, 149–150, 167
Onset, position, quality, quantity, related
    symptoms, setting, transforming
    factors (OPQQRST), 102–106
Open-ended questions
  formulating, 37–38
  health outcomes and, 73
OPQQRST. *See* Onset, position, quality,
    quantity, related symptoms, setting,
    transforming factors (OPQQRST)

P
Paralanguage, 36, 37, 259
Partnership
  shared understanding, 114
Patient-centered care, 142
Persistence
  uncovering theory of illness and, 67
Personal story
  enhance engagement, 17, 18
  obtaining later in interview, 18
  open-ended inquiry and, 18
  relationship to symptoms, 16–17
  time frame, 2, 4, 16
Phases of family interview
  evaluate problem
  identify strengths/resources, 165
  join, 149, 155, 158–160
  organize/contract, 160–162, 166
  plan, 154, 156–158, 160, 165–166

PHQ-9
  screen, 200
Platt, F.W., 17, 32, 35, 57, 80, 88, 229, 252,
    255, 258
Practice, 1–5, 7, 10, 16, 18, 25, 30, 31, 37–38,
    45–48, 50, 53, 54, 63, 66, 73, 78,
    100, 102, 116, 135, 140, 141, 158,
    167, 170, 171, 175, 176, 190–192,
    198, 200, 203, 205, 211, 216, 219,
    237–238
Precision
  vague patients, 90–91, 94
Premature closure
  history of present illness, 100
Preparation, 50, 74, 75, 130, 190–192, 203,
    238, 260
Preschool children
  drawings, 124–125
  play, 125
Progressive structuring
  wandering patients, 79–80, 255, 259
Proxemics, 36, 259
Psychoeducation, 42, 138, 143, 165, 170
Psychosocial issues, 25, 27–28

R
Rapport, 37, 53, 67, 99, 120, 122, 158–160,
    166, 234, 257, 259
Recall errors
  anchor points, 91
  sequencing of events, 91
Referred gate, 71, 72, 78, 116
Reflection, 1–2, 7, 57, 58, 229
Repetitions
  during an interview, 1, 135, 250, 253
Rescuing
  alcoholic families, 8
Restatement, 74, 109, 115–117, 149, 259
Rider, E.A., 125
Risk factors
  suicide, 197, 198, 202
Role play
  contracting, 2, 5, 6, 8, 9, 21–22, 26, 41, 49,
      63, 71, 83, 149, 158, 181, 219, 243
  externalize thoughts of interviewer, 5
  participation, 2, 3, 5, 6, 149, 207, 210
  phobic reaction, 3
  repeat, 3, 7–9, 73, 210, 252
  reverse, 5, 53, 73, 259
  safety, 2–4, 7, 9, 53
  time limits, 7, 198
Rothenberg, M.B., 113, 259
Runaway interview, 80

Rupture repair
  relationship, 253

S
Sadness
  intense, 56, 59–60, 251
Safe environment
  contracting and, 35
  empathy, 36
  listening and tracking, 35
  nonjudgmental, 35
  normalization, 36
School-aged children
  mix of open and closed-ended
      questions, 125
  sense of competence, 125
Secondary data, 101, 107
Selective serotonin reuptake inhibiters
      (SSRIs), 204–205
Self-awareness
  definition, 7, 259
  family-of-origin similarities, 7, 8, 73,
      124, 225
Sensitive topics
  behavioral incident, 91, 93
  denial of the specific, 91, 92
  gentle assumption, 91, 92
  normalization, 91–92
Sequencing of events
  recall errors, 91
Setting the platform in suicide assessments
  establish engagement, 200
  patient in touch with psychic pain, 200
  stay fully present, 200
Sexual history
  adolescents, 211
  adults, 212, 217
  clarifying responses, 217
  clinician's responsibility, 211
  functioning and, 212, 217
  high risk behaviors, 212, 217
  interfering beliefs, 211
  interviewing and, 210
  relationship issues, 211, 212
  setting the stage, 211, 212
Shea, S.C., 4, 36, 38, 77, 91, 199
Shut-down adolescents
  avoid annoyance, 128
  discuss topics of interest, 129
  new contract, 29
  third-person technique, 128
Somatic fixation, 29, 181, 183, 184,
      187, 250

SSRIs. *See* Selective serotonin reuptake
    inhibiters (SSRIs)
Structuring strategies
    contracting, 74, 76
    guiding, 74, 77–79
    make process overt, 74, 76
    preparation, 74, 75
    time management, 74–76
Style of interviewer
    accuracy, 88, 89
Suicide
    contract with primary care clinicians
        prior to, 198
Suicide assessment
    CASE method, 201
    current suicidal episode, 191, 203
    interfering beliefs, 198, 199
    mistakes, 198
    normalization, 200–201
    past suicidal behavior, 191, 200, 202–203
    screen, 135, 191, 200, 201, 203, 205
    sequencing, 191, 201, 202, 205
    setting the platform, 189, 190, 196, 199–200
Symbolic meaning of illness, 68, 69
Synectics, 45

T

Tasks of the interview
    closing phase, 74
    middle phase, 74
    open phase, 74
Think family
    family oriented questions, 146
Third-person technique, 56, 78, 114, 116, 125,
        128, 184, 208, 216, 219, 220, 259
Time management, 73–76
Touch
    empathy, 36
    family members, 159
    runaway patient, 80

Tracking, 8, 13, 21, 31, 35, 41–43, 49, 63,
        64, 71, 76, 80, 83, 89, 93, 96,
        100–102, 110, 129, 153, 159,
        163, 171, 200, 203, 216, 228,
        229, 239, 255, 259
Training in mental health
    primary care and, 170, 174
Transitions
    empathic summaries, 60, 71, 77, 78, 95,
        97, 102, 103, 149, 189
    implied gate, 78
    referred gate, 71, 78
    third-person technique, 78, 216
Trust
    cultural, 143

U

United States Preventive Services Task Force
    (USPSTF), 200, 224
USPSTF. *See* United States Preventive
    Services Task Force (USPSTF)

V

Vagueness
    cognitive deficit, 89–90
    increasing precision, 90–91
Validity
    inquiry into alcohol use, 226
Verbal videotape, 203
Video moments, 46

W

Wandering patient
    progressive structuring, 79, 255, 259
Werewolf, 65, 66
Winging it, 201
Worry
    vs. concern, 55, 258